# The L
# Schizophrenia

## Based On A True Story

# Cory Kaldal

**chipmunkapublishing**
the mental health publisher

Cory Kaldal

Published by
Chipmunkapublishing
United Kingdom


http://www.chipmunkapublishing.com

Copyright © Cory Kaldal 2013

ISBN    978-1-84991-993-7



Chipmunkapublishing gratefully acknowledge the support of Arts Council England.

# Chapter 1

I open the door from my psych ward room in One South in the Kamloops hospital. The clock read eleven after midnight, the lights were low and the nurse asked me what am I doing up? I would have thought the nurse in my situation would understand I couldn't sleep so I replied with a low voice "may I go for a smoke? I cannot sleep". The nurse sighing at me like I was bothering her while she read a magazine says to me "Ok, but you have to be very quiet; you are supposed to be sleeping!" The rules of the back of the psych ward were one smoke an hour, but at this time of night, there was to be no one allowed to be smoking. My doctor had me on Haldol a very old drug which made me very foggy in my head, it also made me walk very slowly. All I could do was shuffle my feet at a very slow pace in the blue polyester slippers. The slippers seemed cheap, there soles made of cloth and only a small bit of Velcro to hold them together. Dr. Alan my psychiatrist put me on Haldol because they needed to start with the oldest drugs and work up to newer ones depending on how I reacted to them. The nurse handed me one of my cigarettes and escorted me quietly to the side door. The nurse smiled at me and said "Be quick dear" and wedged the door behind me. Even though I was at the back end of the psych ward the nurses were kind to me. I reached for my lighter in a slow motion manner and I light the cigarette. I started smoking the cigarette and was noticing it was unseasonable warm out for being a few days away from Christmas. It of course was an El Niño year and it was slightly slushy raining and in my mind it seemed like the sky was melting. Still thinking that this world has ended for me, I cannot shake the feeling of damnation towards my inner soul. Feeling outside of reality as well outside of nature, not feeling human, I wept quietly to myself. I finished the cigarette which seemed to be done just as fast as I light it, I shuffled my feet back into the psych ward and into my room. When I entered the room it seemed illuminated buy a dull glow of orange and red. I looked at the caged window which couldn't be seen from inside to the outside but rather to look into the room from the outside in. I was thinking of my soul on the other side of the window. I was sitting on a wooden chair in a room with no exits and walls of brimstone, I was burning in hell. I crawled back into my bed, fixated on the window and closed my eyes and cried myself to sleep. I awoke to the sound of the breakfast cart the next morning. I crawled out of my bed and sat outside the door in a chair slowly rocking back and forth. I couldn't stand the feeling of sitting nor standing and the only thing to alleviate the sensation of jumping out of my skin was rocking back and forth. There was other people who were admitted to the psych ward eating there food. Breakfast was eggs and sausages; they tasted so good it was amazing as if I never tasted them before. When they took my blood when I was admitted to the psych ward it came back anaemic. I had two helpings of breakfast that morning there was extra food from people in the ward not wanting anything. When I was done breakfast I started my rocking back and forth again in my chair and stared into the linoleum floor. The floor began to melt and I began having images of overwhelming doom, I was tied to a post and in heaven I was being mocked. My brain on fire became like solid dark matter, my eyes froze dark and cold. Then Sandra, a woman I dreamed and longed for, walking up to me smiling said "you will be the only damnation in existence, because of you everyone else will be free to walk in heaven" I began weeping in my chair. Fixated on the floor, watching as the lines began to melt into one another and the desk started to melt unto the floor. A nurse approached me with a smile. "Are you feeling

Better today Ben?" "Fine" I exclaimed. "You're going home today for the holiday's, your mom will be by soon. "Thank you" I said to the nurse as she took the blood pressure machine. I rolled up my sleeve trembling, "This won't hurt a bit" the nurse said softly, as she wrapped the strap around my arm. The nurse pumping the blood pressure cup fast, soon I began to feel the pressure of the strap and a sensation of my eyeballs protruding out of its sockets overwhelming me. Whimpering I was hoping it wouldn't make my head explode. She turned a valve with a hiss, "There, almost done" she said looking at her watch as she took my pulse. Un-strapping me she put back the blood pressure machine and walked back down the hall. The hospital floor gave her shoes clacking sounds of a sharp dull echo as she walked down the hallway. I began to rock slowly again in my chair arms crossed and palms of my hands clutching my elbows. I looked at the clock watching the second hand tick, there seemed to be some meaning to the way it moved with tracers following each tick. Memories of the past week made my stomach feel like it was digesting itself. Flashbacks entered in and out of my visual memory like razorblades on my eyes. Being so overwhelmed with emotions I began to sit up stopping half way from the chair to fully erect debating if sitting down would stop this uneasy feeling of trying to stand. Reconsidering I finished the momentum of standing and began shuffling to the nurses' station. There were other people admitted to the back of One South the same time I was, all for different reasons. Two other people around my age early twenty's to late teens were listening to music and sitting in chairs reading. "May I go for a cigarette please?' I asked the nurse. "Actually Ben" the nurse said in a soft caring voice, "you may go to the lounge and wait for your mom there." " You can go for a smoke if you feel like it from there" she handed me my cigarettes, pointing down the hall and said " just go down the hall past the nurses' station and take a left down that hall you will come to the lounge on your left." Thanking her I began my slow shuffle to the nurses' station. Before I could leave the back of One South I had to walk past the security guard. Shuffling past him I say "Merry Christmas" he smiled and said "Merry Christmas to you too". He was a pretty big fellow considering I was six foot one myself; I seemed to be a lot smaller than him. Then again in my current situation I was mostly skin and bones. I slowly shuffled my feet down the hallway and as I passed by the rooms of the ward I noticed some people were packing to go home others were lying in bed in there room, the sound of Christmas music was getting louder as I passed the nurses' station. I walked past the nurses' station, the nurses doing final release paper work for some of the patients, others getting medications in order, they all seemed busy. Some of them occasionally were glancing at me smiling. I wave and say Merry Christmas as I walked by, the head nurse Elizabeth replied to me "Merry Christmas!" Walking towards the lounge, I seen across from the double doors of the lounge it opened up to the lobby where the entrance to One South was. It was overcast today and the light shone brightly threw the double glass doors and windows. I entered the lounge and seen it was decorated in really old Christmas decorations, there was a stereo on the wall next to the fireplace playing a local radio station. Sofas were on the left side of the lounge next to the fireplace and off to the right were the kitchen and dining area. They had an old fake Christmas tree next to the complimentary caffeine free coffee and bran muffins. Through the door adjacent to the lounge on the right was a fully equipped kitchen with stove, sinks, and microwave. Inside someone was baking fresh chocolate chip cookies, the smell lofting over the fresh brewed decaf coffee was almost overwhelming. Some people were on the sofas reading, in the center of the lounge was a pool table vacant. I was a bit of a shark at pool, it was a pastime that myself and my friends played often. There were a few people at the dining tables talking; some were visiting relatives to admitted patients. In my state of mind having a conversation with anyone would not be more than a few words so I quietly walked to the opposite side of the lounge where the bay doors opened up to the court yard. The courtyard was allocated for people who wished to smoke as I walked outside there was an old tin shed with a table and rickety chairs in it for smokers, when the weather was not so great. There were two elderly ladies in there talking up a storm I asked if I may join them, they said of course. I sat down slowly still having the feeling of jumping out of my skin I reached for my lighter and cigarettes. Both women were wrapped up in there hospital blankets from their beds and I was in my hospital P.J.'s and a robe. I noticed that both women had old hands with terrible nicotine stains on them and nails that looked like they could use a little cleaning. I began to light my cigarette and the lady across from me piped up. "Whenever I have a cigarette I think it's Satan". Thinking to myself maybe I picked the wrong time to sit down, as well the thoughts that floated in my mind I thought inhaling the smoke was going to kill me. She then continued saying "what I like to do is when I butt my smoke I say I am butting you out Satan, Thank you Jesus!" the woman sitting next to me said "yes! Thank you Jesus!" My gut churned of impending doom. Inside the tin shed it had a foul smell, almost like urine and gasoline. It was almost too much to bear; I butted my smoke leavening a huge leftover and said, "I'm butting out Satan I have to go now." I exited the shed as fast as possible thinking ok next time the lesson is don't sit in the shed. Both women continued their discussions of butting out Satan; I went inside and looked for somewhere to sit. There was an open sofa chair next to the fireplace and radio. I began to walk over and I sat down, the chair was unbelievably soft, I sank deep into it. My mind seemed to float in and out of consciousness. The radio was set to 95.3 CJMK. Most the music seemed to be directed at myself and my minds damnation, but then Sandra came on the radio, and I began to weep. The music intoxicates my soul, not an obsession, but a voice in my lonely tormented mind. My existence was meaningless to me; I was nothing more than a wandering soul on the moon of my dreams. I do not exist on earth, but my halo burns its inscription around my brow. My life in my mind seemed like lies I told myself to make me feel something of who I am. I gazed into the lobby and time was no longer with me. Fleeting was the music that ended too soon, and I was left to wonder when her grace would be present again in my soul. Was this my destiny of riddles and secrets I could not utter to anyone? A voice boomed, "Ben!" Echoing threw my body and stopping my heart beating for but a second. I was lost. I closed my eyes and just rocked back and forth biting my lips and my tongue. My body was being torn from all angles of the room. I could not think of more than how my damnation would be only to myself, and all life will be among heaven. I opened my eyes to a voice "excuse me would you like a chocolate chip cookie I just baked them?" "Sure" I said weeping. How does one be happy and sad at the same time? I took one cookie and the girl smiled and walked around the room passing out her fresh cookies. I ate the cookie in desperation and of gratitude towards the act of kindness. Finding it tough to swallow, I walked over to the coffee pot and poured myself a coffee. Looking around I seen there was no cream our sugar, the thought of black coffee made me want to gag. I asked one of the people standing next to the counter by the sink "do you know if there is any cream or sugar?' the man replied "apparently it's against the rules they don't want anyone freaking out on a sugar or caffeine high." "But there's cream in the fridge over there if you would like some." "Thank you" I said to the man and I wandered over to the fridge and found the cream. I quickly poured the cream in my coffee and stirred it with a coffee stir stick. Almost choking from the cookie I slowly drank the hot coffee and began to walk towards the sofa chair. Once my throat was cleared of the cookie I really noticed how disgusting the coffee was that I was drinking. I was slowly shuffling back to my sofa seat I casually walked past the garbage can and shovelled my coffee in it. I noticed a nurse walking down the hall from the nurses' station and into the lounge, she looks around and as I approached she asks, "Are you Ben?" "Yes" I said thinking to myself she must know I'm damned. "We've been looking for you, you need to get your things and get dressed your mom will be here any minute!" she turns around back to the nurses' station and I slowly make my way back to my room. I finally make it to the end of One South as the security guard moves his legs from across the door frame to let me by. Thanking him I make my way into my room and started to get changed. When I emerged from my room I notice the room next to mine off to the left that there's an old lady in it staring at the ground. I walk towards the open door and gesturing my hands together in a preying fashion, I bow. Looking at her I thought she had a very large forehead and I thought to myself that her brain was one big tumor and she belonged to god. Looking up at me with forgetful eyes she murmurs to me "I know why you're here" in astonishment I said softly "you do??" "Yes" she replied, "you're here about my house!" in utter disappointment I thought, why the hell am I standing here like this? I turn around and the nurse telling me as I was leaving the end of One South to go to the lobby my mom was here. I walked down the hall and could see my mom Alice talking to the head nurse Elizabeth. Finally making it to the nurses' station, Elizabeth looks up at me and says "well you're all set to go home for the holidays Ben I hope you enjoy yourself." I replied with a thank you and Merry Christmas. "Before you go Ben you have to sign the in/out log book" I sign the log book and hand it back to Elizabeth. She hands my mom my medication, and we head towards the lobby of one south to go home. I walk through the double doors of One South, my mom was behind me. My parents truck a 91' GMC was on the curb with my step dad Jerry inside waiting for us. I went in the back of the extended cab truck and my mom sat in the passenger seat. We made our way from the hospital which is located down town Kamloops and drove towards the highway. Down the road a ways was my old hang out after I came from work from the night club I worked at. Passing the Breakfast Restaurant their windows tinted, I thought my old buddy Richard Brown was inside disgusted by my damnation and shaming me. The feeling of sorrow was so intent that I was on the verge of tears. Richard was a big fellow but we had good times at Uncle Ralph's the night club both him and myself use to work weekends at. The Breakfast's was a ritual for us after work; we usually sat there till daylight bullshitting about what we had to deal with at work. My mom turns and looks at me. "Were going home Ben then I'm taking you in the car to a doctor's appointment." "Why do I have to see the doctor?' not pleased about the situation. "You're getting a new prescription and we need to talk to him before you come home to stay for the holidays, we also have to pick up grandma." The drive home from the hospital was un-eventful; we lived about fifteen minutes out of town in a suburb called Rayleigh. Pulling into the driveway I could see my grandmother Gene looking out the living room window patiently waiting for us to arrive. I walk into the house and my grandma greats me with open arms giving me a hug. My mother took the car keys as we head back out the door to go to the doctor's appointment. My mom had the radio playing in the car as we drove from the house. Sandra was on the radio, singing. Fear is what I felt. Fear that I will soon die in this world an abomination of god. No one ever tells you that life outside of yourself is a scary place to be. Not knowing what reality is all of an illusion and dreams, the ghosts in my mind did haunt me so. Fearing what I was thinking in my own mind I could not explain to my family how I felt alone in existence a breed apart of life. How I had visions of god and seen him in glory. Feeling joy and then utter despair, I was left outside of heaven. All I heard was the music and I had to ante up to a life I did not foresee. My grandmother turns to me and says "Ben did you know you went missing for four days?" "I did?" I exclaimed in astonishment. My memories were nothing more of a nightmare stretched in fragmented time over a blur of night and day it all seemed like I was among death. "Can you tell me of what happened to you while you were missing?" my grandma tearful with anxiety over the whole ordeal. Shivering and shaking my head I couldn't speak of anything so painful to my soul and so frightening to my inner being all I could do was shake my head and look out the window crying. My grandmother kind enough to realize I was having trouble with my thoughts let me be till we arrived at the doctor's office. Whimpering to my mom and grandma as we sat in the waiting room of the doctor's office I softly spoke to them that I could not talk about what happened. My mother understanding says "its ok Ben we will be your advocate and you don't have to say anything." Dr. Alan walked out the door he was a tall gangly man with a strait narrow face with a dark moustache and goatee and motioned for us to come in, my anxiety and fear overwhelmed me and I slunk in the sofa he had in his office as my mother and grandma sat next to me. Dr. Alan with his straight and narrow face looks at me and says "so Ben how are we doing today?" I was unable to breath, my mother starts explaining to him I'm not doing too well and that they will be speaking on my behalf. Mr. Alan soon explains that it will probably take a year or longer to come to a diagnosis for myself and that even such a diagnosis is not concrete. From what he has seen of me in the psych ward he is leaning towards a schizophrenic diagnosis. The message he had was quite grim. He explained that I could start to drool from my medication and that; it's possible that it would be permanent. He went on to say that a very high percentage of schizophrenics commit suicide. There was also no cure for schizophrenia and he was quite honest in saying they really don't know exactly what it was. Most studies are inconclusive and that what is good for one person is not so good for another. He went on to say there is two types of symptoms to schizophrenia what he called positive and negative. My family was quite upset at what he was saying and had too many questions and worry to think about. "But Ben you don't have to worry about your smoking." "I don't condone smoking." "But most people with Schizophrenia smoke tobacco; even though smoking is harmful it is in this case not a serious cause for concern for now.' He went on to say, "There's something in the tobacco that helps alleviate the symptoms of the illness and symptoms of the medications." "There will be weight gain to the medications all of them have that side effect." "And were going to be trying a new experimental drug with you called Chlomazapene." smiling he says to me "I hope you don't mind being a Guinea pig." chuckling he wrote out the prescription, "I am also prescribing another drug called Lorazopam it helps with anxiety and you should take them twice a day, but there are considered a narcotic and they are highly addictive I would seriously recommend you try and wean yourself from them." With that, he handed my mother the prescriptions, both my grandma and mother thanking him and I began to walk out the door. Dr. Alan handed my mother some sample packs of the new medication and he said I should take it in the mornings and at bedtime. I slowly shuffled my way through the waiting room of the office and we began to get in the car. "We're going to get these prescriptions filled, ok Ben?" my mother explaining. I nodded, and we began to go to the opposite side of town. As we drove my mind wandered over the past week of what had happened, recalling bits of images of my trauma of my psychotic breakdown and being missing for four days I recall the police picking me up in Winfield British Columbia at the seven eleven at five in the morning. Eating cream of wheat in the cell they put me in, the soupy breakfast swirled with the brown sugar in the Styrofoam bowl. Recalling an innocent presence break my soul, like a small sliver in my mind. Crossing the bridge over the Thompson River that divided Kamloops, we headed towards the Grocery Store in north shore. I see blue sky's in the horizon off to the west where the river would meet the Kamloops Lake. Traffic was hectic being a few days from Christmas I had the feeling of nostalgia and a sense that Christmas will never be the same in my life again. My mother expressing subtle similarity's towards my feeling of Christmas she was deeply saddened about my situation. We parked the car in the busy parking lot and my mother ran in to fill the prescription, my grandma let me step outside for a cigarette and there was a cold chill to the breeze that filled the morning. I was in a blue star wars hooded sweater that I had since high school and my grandma asked "are you worried about gaining weight Ben from the medications?" I told her I was willing to let that happen if it meant I could have some form of comfort from fighting myself of anxiety. I of course was built like Athlete from trying to become a full time member of the Kamloops fire department, I was still on my leave of absence to go to school in Vancouver however my situation changed so dramatically that my future in the fire department was not going to happen any time soon. I was going to Vancouver animation school to become a movie board writer and animator, however while attending the school I became ill with a psychotic breakdown that lead me to where I ended up in One South. My mother was coming back to the car as I finished my cigarette and we got in the car deciding to go to the Pancake Palace's across the street from Grocery Store for lunch while we waited for the prescription. The afternoon was starting to warm up and the overcast started to clear slightly and give way to some sun shine. We were seated to an empty table it was quite this afternoon only a handful of people occupied the Restaurant and the waitress came and took our orders. I ordered the grand slam and my mom and grandmother shared chicken strips and fries. Sitting at the table I felt as though the building was leaning in a forty five degree angle as if the earth was tilted and couldn't shake the feeling like gravity was pulling me to one side. My mom and grandma was trying desperately for me to explain to them how I felt and in my mind I felt as though I was struck with a rapture of the mind, if I could put to words my damnation I would, but all I did was shake my head and say I cannot explain it. Soon the food came to our table and I devoured it so fast it was like I never had food before, I finished my plate well before mom and grandma could get there's half finished. Sipping on my coffee while my grandma and mom ate there food I had visions of stars being angels perches in heaven and they would come to earth to kill. My hallo was my prison and my wings were to anchor me like a ball and chain. Out of the corner of my eye I seen a light like a small star drop from the ceiling and when I looked over it was gone only to glance at the table at my coffee cup to see it jump from my cup to the ceiling. Terrified not knowing if what I saw was real my grandma noticed I was agitated and I just shook my head unable to talk about what just happened. My mom sitting across from me asks "can you find some way to tell us what you're going through?" trying to speak me felt that someone had pressed a mute button on my tongue and I slowly murmured the words, "I feel like I want to jump out of my skin." Going on I said, " I feel like the sky is falling, as if a giant anvil or piano is going to fall from the sky and land on me head." My grandma chuckles "Ben, the sky isn't falling and a piano won't fall on your head!" I looked at her as if she was telling me a lie, "How do you know?" I retorted. "Ben!" my mom trying to say sternly while trying to hold back laughing, " Ben, I can guarantee a piano won't fall on your head." thinking to myself they know I'm damned in this life and are trying to trick me, I let the conversation end. "You just need to take it easy for a while Ben, the breakdown was like putting your mind threw a blender." images of my brain in a blender shot threw my visual aspects, and nearly horrified at the thought, I know they could read my mind and I better not say anything else. Anxiety sapped my body like a knife through butter and the dull choking sensation in my throat was hard to take while I was sipping on my coffee. After lunch we left the restaurant and got in the car and drove across the street to the Grocery store. Mom was took some groceries before she got my prescription and something for me to drink so I could take my first pill of the new medication. Both I and my grandma were going to wait in the car while she got what she needed and I was smoking like a fiend in a delusion of sorrow. The nightmares not over and this would be the beginning of a life I never asked for. The reason I wanted a job in the fire department was to help people, but god works in mysterious ways and he had a higher path for me to follow. Not knowing what was next for me, the world was a much scarier place then I have ever felt before. Even though I was terrified, I would never give up on to try and keep going on with my life. What felt like hours waiting in the car, my grandmother Gene and I were growing impatient, "where the hell is your mother?" my grandma muttered I replied "I was thinking the same thing." I was sitting in the back seat with my forehead resting on the front seats head rest. Staring down at my hands I wondered if my hands were the hand of god. 'I see your mother, here she comes!" my grandmother growled with inpatients, my mom had a full grocery cart of white bags full of food." "Ben you better help your mom load those into the car." my grandma growing impatient at sitting for so long while my mom shopped, I could not say I blamed her, sometimes my mom seems like she pokes along while shopping. I got out of the back seat of our Honda Accord and began to unload the groceries in the trunk of the car. My mother handed me a pop to wash down the medicine I was about to take, and she then told me to go take back the cart and get the quarter it takes for using the cart. Driving away from the Grocery Store I could see around Kamloops that the rolling mountainsides were speckled lightly with blotches of snow. The traffic was heavy for Kamloops afternoon tomorrow night would be Christmas Eve and people were bustling around the town trying to get that last bit of Christmas shopping done before the big day. My grandmother handing me a sample pack of medicine from the doctor's office, "here is your medication Ben, now we don't have to think about it the rest of the day." I pop a white pill from the blister pack and wash it down with a Coca-Cola. The sun was already approaching sunset it would get dark early in this part of the world being in the Thompson valley of British Columbia. Driving on the freeway home I begin to feel anxiety overwhelm me and I slip into a flashback of my psychotic episode.

## Chapter 2

A fountain of slushy snow and mud slammed my car windshield as I drove up the Coquihalla; semi-trucks were no mercy going past my little 83 Honda civic. The force of the mud and wet snow nearly sending me off into the shoulder, driving to the summit of the high way, my engine screaming as I tried to keep pace with traffic. The sky was clear with a full yellow moon shining through the mountainside trees. Flicking my wiper blades to wipe the mud and snow from my windshield, I noticed I was out of windshield wiper fluid, my mind on fire with visions of going over the embankment and being buried in snow. Only to be found by wolves and bears gnawing at my flesh. Seeing the stars through the side window I would gaze up and see that my life will soon end. A light from my dashboard glowed a pale orange E. I laughed and thought now I am a blaze from the sun; my soul glowing was as hot as the sun itself. Driving up the high way my car started to kick and sputter, in the distance I could see the lights of the summits toll booths. The demons in my head were screaming about my death and I was unsure of how I was going to make it home in the barren snow dead. Visions of me walking on the side road with the trees covered in white snow all that was left was a creature that would devour my soul coming for me. How could I make it home before being devoured by darkness? Approaching the toll booth I began to think I be better off hitch-hiking my way back home, someone in a big truck would pick me up. I began watching semi-trucks drive off in the opposite directions. There were two cars ahead of me going through the toll and approaching the gates I heard voices saying "your life is over! You are nothing more than lies!" rolling down my mud caked window the toll booth attendant looks at me and I ask. " Can you break a big bill?" she looks at me and says "

Depends how big it is" I reach in my pocket and pull out a twenty, the attendant rolls her eyes, she hands me back a ten dollar bill and says thank you. Then I emotionally break down and put the car in reverse and park off to the side of the toll booth building next to the staff parking stalls. I turn off the engine to my car and sit there and have a cigarette. The wall of snow that was put there from the snow ploughs at the edge of the parking stalls was lit up by the toll booths florescent lights. Staring at the snow I imagined walking over the embankment and letting nature do the deed of killing me by being devoured by wolves and bears. The thought of being consumed alive made my heart sink and desperation came over me that I wasn't ready to die yet. I then take my attention to my muddy passenger's seat floors. The floor mat covered in dirt I reach down and find a penny, cleaning it off with my fingers I place the penny in my mouth and set it on the tip of my tongue. With the penny at the tip of my tongue I extend my tongue in my mouth to touch the roof of my mouth with the penny. In a vision I feel my mind go solid as dark ice and my eyes black over with the cold. Envisioning my mind was like one big nuclear bomb about to set off and take out the toll booth and half the side of the mountain in a panic I spit out the penny. Watching all the trucks come out of the toll booth, the toll looking like it was about to fall off the cliff of the side of the mountain, I imagined hitching a ride with a friendly truck driver to my home in Kamloops. Thinking there are no friendlier people other than truck drivers, I step out of my car into the cold night's air. Getting out of my car, the florescent lights nearly blinding me I notice there's another car pulling up next to mine. The car was a beat up Toyota hatchback covered in rust blotches and painted green and yellow. The paint job almost looked like he hand bombed it with aerosol paint cans. I walk over to the passenger side of the car and the driver steppes out of his car.

Looking rather scruffy with beady eyes and glasses, he had a few weeks of bearded growth and a brown toque on. I ask him "where you headed?" "Winfield" he replied, "I'm headed to Kamloops can I hitch a ride?" "Sure, but we don't have any money for the toll" he exclaimed. Digging in my pocket I hand him the ten I had, throwing my car keys on the driver seat of my car. I was expecting to get inside; stopping me he began to clear out the back seat of his car. Thinking I was getting in the back seat I seen him try and pile all the crap he had in his car to the driver's side back seat. I retract the passenger's seat to get in the back; stopping me he pauses then slams the seat back to its original position and gestures for me to get into the passenger seat in the front. I get in and begin to light a smoke, "is it ok I smoke in the car?" "No" he says. "It's ok ill just roll down the window a crack and you won't notice it" I said, and continue to light the cigarette. We go through the toll booth and start down the highway of snow and mud; I look up at the pale yellow moon and then fixate my eyes on the dashboard of the car. Above the glove compartment there was an inscription in quotes written in white out blotches. The inscription read "The Lord is my Rock" and flooded with images of myself in the middle of the ocean sitting on a giant rocky iceberg came over me like a jolt. I look up at the moon and say in a small whisper, "you shall not find me." Like a knife gouging my heart, the memory shaming me in the moment of anxiety, my grandmother turns around and tells me "were home Ben." I open my eyes to see that we are pulling into the carport. The carport was half full with dry wood logs for our wood stove we had in the basement, to heat the house over the winter. At the end of the long pile of wood was my Honda civic which looked like its seen better days and could really use a good wash. I step out of the car and my mom opens the trunk and I began the deed of unloading all the groceries into the house. I walk into the basement and see it's refurbished into a day-care for children. My mom had started her home job with the day-care few months after I left for Vancouver animation school. I take a look round and see she had my star trek model of the star ship voyager sitting high on one of the shelves. There was a large round table the height for children with several small blue chairs around it. Steffi's and toys were to the side in a box next to the TV. My mom had books and her filing cabinet in the back. The entire room looked like a small pre-school. Alice pipes up and says. We moved you to the far room upstairs Ben, grandma is now in your old room in the basement. "We have a few kids coming tomorrow Ben while their parents finish working for the holidays." my mom trying to explain to me. I took as many grocery bags as I could carry and take them upstairs to the kitchen. I heave the bags onto the counter and walk into the dining room; looking out the sliding glass doors I see the mountain near the freeway was bare of snow. Going from the dining to the living room which was adjacent with no walls the Christmas tree was decorated next to our forty five inch projection TV. That was the Christmas present my step dad Jerry bought for my mom for Christmas. My grandma talking from the kitchen "See how big the TV is Ben?" " you should of seen Jerry and your brother bring it in, they had to get Dan for help!" now it wasn't that Jerry and Steve my brother and Dan were weaklings, it was the fact the TV stood about four and a half feet from top to bottom all solid wood and screen. The freaking TV must of weighed close to three hundred and fifty pounds and was awkward bringing it up through the narrow two flights of stairs to the living room. The living room was filled with decorations and it smelled of lavender and roses from the scented candles my mom had on the coffee table. They had Purdy's chocolates on the coffee table and seeing those I opened the box and snatched a couple. "Where is the computer?" I asked my mom. "It's down stares in Steve's room, but the internet isn't working." The computer was an old IBM one fifty from Radio Shack and our internet was fifty six K dial up. I go downstairs to my brother's room which was opposite side of the day-care and see the computer next to the wall. I sit in front of the monitor and start to stare at my feet. I begin to vision that I am on board the voyager star trek ship and that everyone I know is the crew. My left shoe was the left foot of god and my right shoe was the right foot of god, everyone in my mind began laughing. Leaning back in the chair I tilt my head back and begin to swivel the chair in a continuous motion counter clockwise. Visioning flying through space in my space ship I began to laugh uncontrollably. Thinking to myself that my left foot is evil and my right foot is good I ponder why I'm twirling in the chair and wonder where I could go to keep my path to god on the straight and narrow. After staring at a blank computer screen for several minutes I decide to go upstairs and watch some TV. Several hours had passed since I had taken my medication and I felt extremely exhausted. It was five thirty pm and I wandered into the kitchen to where my mother Alice was making dinner. Asking if I could go to bed, hungry and tired my head felt like a lead weight. Looking at Alice she looks at the time and says "no, it's almost dinner time you can't go to bed yet." Dinner was going to be spaghetti and meat sauce, feeling like I would pass out any moment I sat on the rocker sofa in front of the TV and tried to keep my eyes open. The feeling of throwing up and my head exploding I began to weep in the chair. Gene had light some of the scented candles and the lights were dim, she was watching candid camera. Watching the show I felt as though the hosts were my alter personalities and the videos of people was different personalities of my family and friends. Laughing at the comedy I was sure I would be famous from this show. The psychic link I had with this show made me feel I could travel through where I existed in the real world to the existence of the TV dimension. I could do anything on TV and it was my super power, I was becoming a super hero. Pretty soon the hosts of candid camera started to say exactly what I was thinking and their voices echoed in my mind. Soon a great paranoia set in, thinking my mind was an open book everyone around the world could telepathically link to my mind. I began to have visions of heaven seeing a bright sun shining in the sky I imagined it was the end of the world. I existed through the ages of time an immortal. I was surrounded by other immortals. The time came for us to return to the source of creation. We began to walk over the ocean holding hands in the winds of a hurricane we formed a circle. Life on earth was evolving back to the ocean and together the immortals descended into the depths of the ocean. The pressure of the oceans turned the immortals into microscopic beings of light. But there was something greater in the ocean other than immortals, something that froze them in place in a tomb of darkness. It was the great albino amoeba, devouring the immortal souls and forever imprisoning them. We all were reaped as trophies of a begotten age in time, forever displayed on the mantle of the albino amoeba. " there is only one big fish in the sea" Blinking I jolt in the chair, standing up I head to the washroom crying, my grandma concerned followed me and asked what was wrong? Then from the amoeba I was stricken with a vow of silence, and my mind was quiet and dull. Mouthing an explanation and shaking all I could do was tremble and say nothing. After getting a hold of myself with the amoeba looming in my mind I went back to the rocker sofa and explained to my grandma I was ok, I began to rock in the chair unsure of what reality I was in. Looking out the bay window of the living room I could see the street lamp with a dull orange glow in the winter's darkness, and flakes of white began to fill the orange light.

"Ashes of doom and cinder" I murmured, not sure if I should keep my eyes open or shut, it didn't really matter for I was not in reality, and regardless I still seen the visions. Dinner was very tasty; we had garlic bread with the spaghetti and salad. I thought that I was a holy being and breaking the garlic bread was of great significance. This dinner would be my last supper, before I ascended into heaven as an immortal. While I ate my dinner I imagined I would go into my room and burst into a light being, I would then travel to the ethereal of heaven and left in my wake a shadow that would forever be ablaze in my room of my wings and body. After dinner I went to the bay window and could see the snow falling more heavily, the driveway was slowly becoming covered in the white flakes. I sat on the sofa floating in and out of consciousness. Begging my mom to let me go to bed her finally agreed and I began to edge my way to my room. I crawled into my freshly made bed and tried to lay my head on my pillows, not sure why my head rested an inch above the pillows and with all my effort my head would not completely rest on the pillow. I began to watch my digital clock, it read seven thirty five, this was obviously a code for me to decipher. The two dots pulsating between the seven and three I thought to myself how entertaining it was to watch them pulse. Imagining I was in my grave a tomb on top a mountain side. Giant Psychic spiders began feeding on my soul. Feeling the life of my soul leave me I was sapped in my bed waiting to die. From staring into the darkness my eyes were on fire with the sound of the snow and wind I slowly began to fall asleep. I open my eyes and the clock reads for fifty eight, my head still an inch above the pillow I began to get up. Taking some loose fitting sweat pants and a sweater I walk down the hall from my room and sit on the couch looking out the window. Still dark outside the snow was coming down very hard almost blizzard like. Closing my eyes a few times my eyeballs rolling to the back of my head I slipped in and out of a dream state. Not sure what to do with myself I decide to make a pot of coffee. Bustling around the kitchen I could hear Gene clamour up the stairs. "What are you doing up Ben?" "I can't sleep" looking like I drowned in my blankets Gene began to make some toast and she decided to sit up with me until I was going to try and go back to bed. "If we went for a walk Ben would you go back to sleep?" Gene asked hopping the walk would help. I said sure wanting to walk in the thick snow we bundled up with coats and gloves and toque's, and began to head out the basement door. Heading outside I could see our driveway covered in two feet of snow, the road unploughed we began our walk in the early morning blizzard. Treading the deep snow we only walked a few blocks before turning around home, snow falling from the street lamps and whisking along the over flow of the roads. It was almost peaceful being in the blizzard like songs sweet melody of a winter's night, the darkness gave me comfort to my inherent psychotic thoughts. Brushing off the snow in the carport grandma motioning to take a few pieces of wood for the wood stove, I took the wood and taking off my coat and mittens I open the wood stove to see white ashes of the previous wood. Taking some newspaper I start the fire in the stove after filling it with wood and I leave the door to the stove slightly open creating a vacuum. Soon the dry wood was on fire and the oven was being super-heated from the doors vacuum. Closing the door the flames would die down to a smoulder. Slowly warming the house I decided to return upstairs and make myself a coffee. Gene followed me and we entered the kitchen our faces still wet from the snow outside. Mixing three teaspoons of sugar and cream into my coffee I jump up on the counter and sit, swinging my legs back and forth. Thinking I jumped up to heaven and my feet dangled in the glory of the earth it was a hell of a long way back down to where I came from. Perched on my pedestal I would flex my back to hear my angelic wings flutter in the ethereal winds of the soul. Gene looking at me wondering what I was thinking began to talk about how awful it was when I was missing she went on to say that she sat by the phone sick hopping they would find me. I explained how scared I was but I couldn't explain why I was scared or why I went off missing, I said to her ' It was something that I just had to do." confused my grandma started to change the subject towards my mother's day-care how she was having two babies come today, and they are loud criers. It was going to be a short working day for my mom the parents of the children only worked for a few hours today and that the babies would mostly be napping after they ate lunch so we probably wouldn't see much of them. Gene went into the living room and lit the scented candles. I asked "why are there so many candles?" Gene replied "we have them so you can find your way home." In awe at the statement I thought how lost I was and if the nightmares would ever end. I decide to lie on the sofa watching the candles, Gene took one of her scandal magazines and took a pen to do the crosswords, and soon I began to drift off to sleep. Waking to a door slamming and babies crying I was left groggy from waking up, feeling like I must of drank five cases of beer the night before. The medication I had taken the previous day was becoming horridly like a very big hang over. My eyes aching to the light of the overcast sky snow was lightly sputtering down nowhere near the downfall of this morning. I began to light a cigarette and just before I light it, Gene says "you can't smoke in the house anymore Ben it's not good for the kids" "if you want to smoke you have to go on the patio, you can't go in the carport while the kids are here", I walk into my bedroom and take an old sweater and walk towards the patio door next to the kitchen. Taking my smokes I head out the door. The cool crisp air was refreshing the house from the wood stove made it overly stuffy. Looking at the mountainside the mountain was covered in white silky snow, the cloud line was close to the top of the mountain, and then the morning sun cut threw an opening in the clouds and a beam of light shown on the mountainside. Bright orange line sat on the mountainside like the line of a pupil of a cat's eye. The clouds around the beam of sunlight shown orange and I could see lightly flaking snow coming from the west horizon to the side of the mountain off to the east. The message to me from god was the light represented my soul on fire, and I would be marked in this life as an angel of god. Finishing my smoke I walked into the dining room to see my mom getting the high chairs for the two babies so they could eat their lunch. Mom was making spaghetti-O for the children's lunches. My mom went down stairs to take the two babies and put them in their high chairs, there was a boy and girl, the boy's name was Bowden and the girls name was Britney. Bowden was crying up a storm, then my mother handing me the boy said "hold him while I get Whitney in her high chair". When Bowden was in my arms he took hold of my arm looked at my mom and slammed his head on my chest, stopping his crying he looked tired. My mom laughing took him and put him in the high chair. Bowden fascinated with me would be talking his goo-goo and pointing at me. Mom laughing started to feed them both the spaghetti-O. The little tykes ate there food almost as fast as I eat mine when I'm hungry. Before they knew it they ate the whole pot of spaghetti-O. my mom begins taking Bowden out of the high chair and hands him to me, Bowden looking at my mom slams his head on my chest. My mom laughs and says "He likes you Ben, usually he screams before his nap". Smiling, my mom takes Whitney out of the high chair and I follow mom down the hall to the spare room to put the children down for their nap. I decided to sit on the sofa next to the bay window and watch life go bye. My grandma was watching her daytime soap operas and I began thinking of living in the TV, how all their ideas came from my brain. My mother lighting the scented candles and began to crochet a blanket, she was starting this year to finish about twelve of them to donate them to the homeless shelter in town. The city was beginning construction of a new homeless shelter and my mother wanted nice new crocheted blankets on twelve of the beds. Before we knew it, it was three thirty p.m. and Bowden mom drove into the driveway. My mom went into the spare room and woke up Bowden, still sleeping as she carried him in her arms; his mother took him from my mom's arms and began smothering him in kisses. Bowden's mother Kristy wasn't much older than me and she was a very cute woman. Her husband she told me was trying to become a fire fighter and was an auxiliary fire-fighter where I was stationed at when I was in the auxiliary fire department. Embarrassed I wondered what my mother told them of why I was home sick, hopping that they didn't know much my mom stated she never really told her anything when she was leaving. Psychosis was hard thing to describe to people; unlike cancer or breaking your arm psychosis isn't something you can tell someone has other than irrational behavior. Alice told me that she wouldn't disclose why I was sick she never felt it was any of the parents business, although some of her parents wouldn't understand there was one parent who completely understood what it was about, her brother who was twenty was diagnosed with schizophrenia a year before I was. Amy wasn't going to be coming with her children till after the holidays, but my mom was eager for me to meet her. I went upstairs with my mother and we sat in front of the TV on the sofa back to what we were doing before. While watching TV and waiting for Whitney to wake from her nap I looked out

the window and seen a car pull into the drive way, it
was a small red Honda hatchback. I knew who the car
belonged to one of my old friends Chelsea Andrews.
Excited to see a friend I let in Chelsea in from the front
door. The best description for Chelsea was that she
was gorgeous; she was a spitting image of a young
Catherine Zeta Jones. Giving me a big hug when I
opened the door I escorted her upstairs and we began
to chat. One of my favorite past times was going for
coffee with my friends being Christmas Eve I asked my
mom if I could go for coffee. Hesitant at the request my
mom agreed to let me go but not for long we were
having Chinese food for dinner tonight and my brother
would be coming home soon with his girlfriend. I took a
couple packs of cigarettes and made sure I was in
jeans and a good looking sweater. Chelsea was
wearing a tight black skirt and a blouse covered by a
white knitted sweater. I was flirting and I was laughing
as we left the house, she was almost like a dream I
had. I jumped into her car and rolling down the window
I light a cigarette and she was very excited to see me
she heard I went missing and concerned she had to
see me when she knew I was not in the hospital.
Thinking I was the same old Ben she once
remembered she was not prepared for what I was
experiencing with my psychosis. We drove down the
highway to town and I felt so high on life it would be the
first encounter where being in control of my mind was
not going to be the case. Excited to see me, Chelsea
drove down the freshly ploughed highway. She began
to tell me how she had a nightmare the night before of
a demon trying to kill her. Shocked I said how scary
that must have been for her. Then I began to explain
what it was like for me with the visions I was having
and how I felt one with god and soon I would be in the
realm of heaven. Empathizing with me she was
probably more terrified at what I went through then
about her dream being killed by a demon. Driving to

town we decided to have coffee at the restaurant near the first intersection of the freeway coming from Rayleigh. We were seated at a table with a window looking through the Thompson valley. When we sat down she opened her mouth and showed me that one of her teeth had fallen out and a new tooth was growing in its place. Feeling misplaced by how odd it was I said to her laughing, " you must be a vampire" "I know" she laughed continuing on with her story about how she felt like she was five years old again losing her baby teeth. Sipping my coffee I was lightly listening to the radio's music and predicted to her that Sandra would be the next singer on the radio. Sure enough one of her newly released songs was playing. Astonished at my prediction Chelsea asked me how I knew it would be her, smiling I said "that's one of my secrets I've learned how to do lately," Thinking Chelsea will understand when the world dies and heaven will be born unto earth. I drank my coffee fast and watched the cars float by along the freeway. I began to say "I think we should get going Chelsea, dinner will be soon." I paid for our coffee and we left the restaurant smiling and joking to one another. While we drove back to my home, I began to explain how this was meant to be, how today a perfectly in sync day it was. Just before arriving in the suburb of Rayleigh, I looked out the window towards the mountains, and suddenly from my bowels I began to laugh hysterically, a dark and booming laughter. Chelsea terrified tried to make the situation like it was nothing out of the ordinary and says to me. " That's what the demon sounded like in my dream" continuing with the laughing I say to her " See how perfect the day is, I think I'm going to go for a drive when you take me home." she replied that it would be a great idea I do that. Thanking her for taking me for coffee I waved goodbye as she left to go to town. Wondering why I was laughing I went inside and began to look for my car keys. Thinking nothing of it I told my mom I was going for a drive, my mom nearly screaming at me saying "No you are not, being on the medication your on and its almost dinner time we ordered Chinese food already!" she took the keys from my hand and I light a smoke only to put it out and relight it again. After going through nearly a whole pack of smokes relighting and butting them my mom angry says to me " I think your smoking too much Ben!" snatching my pack before she could take them we both felt a level of anger in us. I looked in the pack of smokes and seen I was nearly out wondering how I would get the next pack I reasoned with Alice that ill slow down but I need to go to the store to buy more cigarettes. "We will go to the store after dinner and you can get your smokes." both myself and my mom calming down. My brother Steve and his girlfriend Rena walked up the stairs. Rena was living with us while Steve went to college, Steve was training with his boxing coach he had a tournament at the end of January. Both Steve and I trained in kick boxing while I was working at Uncle Ralph's, the nightclub I use to work weekends at. Steve however was smaller than me however he knew how to throw the punches, I was more power being physically bigger than him, but my brother was more patient. Jerry both I and Steve's step dad rolled in the driveway with dinner and Alice told us to go help him bring it in. Finishing dinner I went to the sofa next to the bay window and began to rock back and forth, anxiety filling me it felt like the house was upside down. Not knowing what to do with myself I felt like standing and sitting as if I was jumping out of my skin, the same feeling like I had while in the psych ward. Panic attacks were common occurrences while dealing with my psychosis, and when my mother seen I was being agitated with my emotions and thoughts she would get a glass of water and hand me a Lorazapam. After washing down the little white two milligram pill, it was almost an instant effect of calming from the drug; it also made me feel sleepy after I consumed it. Feeling my brow burn from my halo, I begged my mom if we could go for a walk outside, nodding my mom took some money and said 'Let's walk to the corner store for your smokes Ben." Taking our winter coats and gloves we headed outside already dark, the fresh air and the night sky gave me a sense of comfort. We walked past the elementary school that was a few houses down from our house and turned up the street crossing the rail road tracks. Wondering if there was actually a train coming at the very moment I was walking across the tracks, one of Jerry's trucker friends Wayne Gorham ran up to my mom gave her a hug and shouted "MERRY CHRISTMAS Alice!" Laughing my mom said merry Christmas and waited for me to catch up to her asking Wayne how he was doing over the holidays. "I'm getting drunk and I don't give a damn!" replied Wayne as he began to walk to his home. Wayne Gorham lived on the other side of Rayleigh, near the Fraser River. Feeling awkward I walked past him and the store just off to the left we began to continue towards the store. Walking into the store Blain an old high school buddy was filling his beater truck with gas. Blain was known as a scrapper in high school and when I first moved to Rayleigh we had our scraps. Later we became good friends and partied every weekend in Rayleigh. There wasn't much for teenagers to do in Rayleigh, other than to cause trouble and get drunk or stoned out of our minds. I pick up two packs of Dry Malls and I see Ryan Ford in the store, Ryan was the Fire Chief where I worked as an auxiliary at Station twenty one. Ryan shaking my hand "don't worry Ben your still on your leave of absence." "I plan on coming back sometime Ryan just not sure when." "There's no rush Ben your good for a few years." little did I know Ryan probably didn't want me to come back for a couple of reasons, one being I failed the pee test just before I was about to be hired for a full time job in the fire department and second he more than likely knew I was in the hospital in the psych ward. While in the fire department I was very responsible and professional, but once I failed the pee test and ended up in the psych ward, I was no longer considered to be respected enough as a member more of a bad blemish in the department that they wanted nothing to do with. Ironically if it was an injury in the department or something other than psychosis I probably would have been given more respect in the department. When I was an auxiliary, one of the fire fighters in station twenty one got in a car accident, the station held a dance / fund raiser for him. Because I failed the pee test and was in the psych ward there was no fund raiser for me, no dance, I was more of a disgrace then anything. Little did I know while talking to Ryan, that I was being segregated and stigmatized? This would not be the last time it would happen. I never did mention to anyone in the fire department of what happened, I didn't have to everyone knew. After realizing this, my career as a fire fighter ended. Walking home from the store I felt as though I was never going to be able to redeem who I was that during my psychosis the person I once knew did in fact die. The person who once was the life of the party with my friends and a responsible person pursuing a great career, died on the cold icy road home, that night on the Coquihalla. It was ironic really the fact I not only felt apart from humanity from being ill but little did I know society itself was placing me in a category of being inhuman. I watched TV for a while hallucinating and seeing my existence being lived out threw the variety of comedy shows. Exposed I felt the world was writing me in a fate I never wanted. I went to bed feeling the psychic spiders feeding on me, my muscles and tendons had the sensation of unravelling in my body. I watched the code on the clock the pulsing double dots seemed to sooth my frustrated mind. Lost I fell asleep in a daze of fog from my night medication. During the night I had a dream, restless I found myself standing in darkness, then in the darkness there was a being that seemed like he didn't belong on this earth, realizing how vivid this dream was I awakened paralyzed. Hearing a strange chatter, heard drills coming towards me. Face in my pillow I could not move screaming I felt the drills in my back. The more I struggled to awaken, the faster the drills would leave holes in my back, beings of darkness stood around me. Trying to move my arms, I felt the drills in my mouth drilling my teeth, flashing in light I wake up in my bed feeling as though I had a hangover, my head pounded with pain every time my heart would beat. Exhausted and unable to sleep I slowly crawl out of my bed. Sliding along the walls of the hallway, I hold my head with palms around my temples. I stumble to the sofa rocker and rock back and forth slowly crying at the pain. Slipping back into dream I feel the eyes of beings not of the earth watching me, little did I know hours had passed which felt like moments and I tried so hard to open my eyes, all I felt was a burning sensation in my legs my knees on fire from not moving in the rocker chair. Waking up to daylight it was Christmas day. My mom waking up began to make pancakes and eggs. I felt like a train had run over me, and began to cry not knowing what to do. I began to walk in a circle from the kitchen to the dining room into the living room back to the kitchen, it felt unbelievably soothing. Alice unsure what I was doing I repeated this clockwise motion all day long. Christmas day passed by with more of uneasy feelings and sadness due to me being ill and lost in psychosis. The nightmare continued that night with the out of body experiences this time I felt my body being pulled through my bedroom walls and leaving me float on the other side. The next day I sat in the sofa rocker in the living room crying, my grandma asking me if my head hurt. "Yes" I said, my grandma walking behind me began to massage my head. Talking to Alice my grandma went and took her blood pressure machine. I unwilling to take my blood pressure they insisted I take it. Feeling like my eyes were bulging, my grandma and mother wondered if it was broken, giving a reading that would have given me the same state as someone having a stroke they began to panic. Today was Boxing Day and they desperately phoned our family Doctor. His last name was Slanders My mom pleading with the receptionist of the doctor's office of what my blood pressure was, Dr. Slanders explained to my mom if she brings me into the office they would phone the police. Angry my mom slammed down the phone and we gathered some clothing and began to head to the emergency room of the Kamloops hospital. Jumping in the car my mom and grandma shoving my backpack in the back seat next to me, they race to Kamloops emergency room. When we arrive I'm escorted to one of the beds and told to sit in the chair my mom leaves to talk to a nurse, and I cross my arms with palms of my hands on my elbows rocking in the chair. Looking at my worn out shoes I vision myself back in my spaceship flying through space, everyone wanting to go somewhere new in the heavens and I was immortal. Patiently waiting at what seemed like hours my mom came back to tell me they had to wait for me to be assessed by a mental health nurse and I would be getting a new family doctor. I was sitting in the emergency room and a nurse came and escorted my mother Alice and myself to a room adjacent to the emergency ward. In the room was a brown chair that resembled a dentist's chair. He nurse pointing to it says to me "you can sit there Ben" thinking the hospital was traveling through space and time I began to feel gravity shift in different directions. With my eyes rolling to the back of my head, I couldn't tell if the hospital was sideways upside down or right side up. Growing impatient and getting dizzy I asked mom when can we leave, stopping me from getting up off the chair said "just wait here I'll go see when the doctor will be here." Finally after what seemed like an eternity my mom walked into the room with our new family doctor, "Ben this is Dr. Sadden" my mother introducing me. Dr. Sadden was a tall man with blonde hair and glasses, his hair looked like he had slept in it and in places was sticking up here and there. I thought Dr. Sadden was an un-dead zombie who before he died was in a car accident where his hair was messed up and sticking out that is where the glass of the windshield stuck in his head. Asking me several questions on how I felt if I was thinking anything out of the ordinary Dr. Sadden asks me "Do you know why you're here Ben?' I say "yes, my mom is trying to kill me" nearly jumping from her chair my mom says " No I'm Not Ben!" after stating that Dr. Sadden seemed to be done with the questions and he walked outside in the hallway with my mom. Soon I was being escorted back to One South. Upon entering one south it seemed to be different it was a lot noisier then when I was there before, could hear people in the lounge talking very loudly almost like the presence was of a demonic power. Walking past the nurses' station I seen Dr. Alan talking with the nurses, apparently the psychiatric doctors would rotate shifts of being the head doctor in the facility. Walking towards the back ward I saw a young security guard who reminded me of a younger version of my uncle Robert. The nurses at the counter of the back ward handed me my hospital attire and said to me " you can go change in the bathroom Ben." after I had gotten changed my step father Jerry was standing with me while my mom went into one of the rooms to talk with Dr. Alan. The nurse at the counter started to talk to me "Ben I need to have your cigarettes you know the rules here!" handing her my cigarettes I walk back to where Jerry was standing and I lean over to him and whisper, " man they sure take things seriously here." Jerry starting to chuckle at that statement, my mom walking towards me wondering what was so funny. Dr. Alan asked to speak with me and walking in the room he explained I would be on new medicine I would take once a day, it was an experimental drug called Risperdal. He was starting me on a very low dosage of one milligram and would increase it over time to see if I would balance out. My family gave me hugs and left to go home leaving me in the care of the hospital. I wasn't in the same room as before they had new people in the back ward, an elderly man named Earl was in my old room he had Alzheimer's and was going to be placed in a care facility. I sat down in one of the chairs next to my room rocking in the chair, the nurse said to me "you just got here in time Ben, the lunch cart should be here shortly" looking down the hall I could see on the ceiling half chrome domes, I knew they were for cameras but I could see red lasers coming out of them. Where ever I looked I could see a red dot then it would vanish. Look at a nurse and glimpse a red dot and then it would vanish. Shaking my head it felt more of an obsessed disorder of seeing the red dots then actually seeing them. Kind of like the obsession is what fuelled me to see lasers. Rocking back and forth looking at the linoleum floor I could see it swirling and moving in waves around my feet, looking back down the hallway hoping I wouldn't see any more red dots the lunch cart was half way down the hall way appearing from nowhere. Wondering what was for lunch today I began to grow impatient. The nurse soon dragged the lunch cart towards the back of the ward not until she stopped at every room that had someone in it. While the cart crept closer to the back ward I saw that people in the back where I was were sitting in chairs next to their room waiting for lunch. With a clunk of the weight of the cart going past the door frame of the backwards double doors; the nurse began to hand out lunch we were the last people to eat. Lunch was a small bowl of chicken noodle soup with a whole wheat sandwich which consisted of ham and butter and tomato. The food was a lot blander then I remember when I was in the psych ward before. Watching Earl he was muttering some strange language and eating hooting once in a while, but otherwise he was pretty calm. After lunch was over the cart rolling back down the hallway I asked if I could go for a cigarette. The nurse obliged and a young man in his twenties wanted to join me. His name was Rick and he began telling me he was here because he attempted suicide. Feeling sick over the reason, he began to explain to me he had issues with bi-polar disorder. He reminded me a lot of my brother I thought this person deserves to be respected as a human being. Even though Steve was my younger brother I looked up to him in a lot of ways. Seeing Steve in Rick it almost brought me to tears that anyone besides me should be here in the psych ward. We light our cigarettes and began talking of how we ended up here, looking down I seen in the bushes something slowly moving, then out of the slimy mud there was a salamander. Laughing at how peculiar a salamander would be in the mud this time of year, Rick went in to show the nurse and the nurse came out and thought it was amazing. After watching the salamander do salamander things it slowly crawled back in the mud and was gone. When went back inside Rick asked If I wanted to have a game of Chess. Remembering the First time I played chess was with my friend Shaun Strode. He used to live in an apartment near the college in Kamloops, and the first summer after graduation of high school we partied and played chess. It had taken me the entire summer to learn how to play well and after a few months I was actually able to beat Shaun at chess. Ever since then chess was something I loved to do as a past time. Rick set up the board on a small table that was in the back ward. We had a few games I lost every time, I knew the fundamental rules of the game and how the pieces worked but I wasn't that good at openings or middle game tactics yet. After a few more games Rick decided he wanted to go into his room and listen to music, I was getting quite tired of playing and thought I'd take a nap in my room. Walking into my room I decided to set my back against the wall with my arms out and palms down on the wall, feeling like I was laying down on the wall and the room was upside down, I watched the sheets on my bed as the morphed and melted into one another, closing my eyes I could feel psychic energies come from the room adjacent from me going into the palms of my hands. With a calming sensation over me I fell asleep leaning on the wall. Dreaming I was floating in the sky and the presence of old friends who were not in this lifetime I landed in my body with a thud. Slamming my feet down I thought I was just in heaven and I came back to earth. Rubbing my eyes I walked out of my room to see the med cart there, it was time for us to take our medications. Everyone lined up to the med cart and one at a time we were handed some water and our medications in a white paper cup. I asked the nurse if I could phone home, the nurse smiled at me and handed me the phone. Calling home I asked when they were coming back to the psych ward, my mom saying we would be there after they had dinner, I asked if she could bring me Restaurant food, a burger and fries maybe? Then I looked at the people in the psych ward and thought if I had something that good they would kill me, so I changed my mind and thought I should wait for the hospital food. Doctor Alan came down to the end of the psych ward and says to me "good news Ben, tomorrow were moving you into the front of the psych ward." thinking to myself thank god these rooms suck. Watching him head back down the hall to the nurses' station, the laser beams no longer beaming, I think well... now what does an angel of god do? I sit in the Chair listening to the beeping of intercoms and I could hear the bustle of the front of the ward with a crash and clank I see the dinner cart come around the nurses' station. Feeling hungry I hopped dinner would be good. Getting my meal I seen it was some sort of mystery meat in a week tomato sauce with vegetable barley soup and a bun and vanilla pudding. Trying to eat the meat it was tough and filled with gristle. Looking at the cart there was a lot of people not eating dinner tonight, someone screaming in the front ward "What is with this Shit for dinner!" I asked the nurse "is it ok if I have other peoples soup and buns and vanilla pudding?" the nurse saying "Sure you can Ben it's just going into the garbage once it leaves here" helping myself to four servings of soup buns and pudding I was in heaven. Vegetable barley soup is one of my favorites, and I scoffed it down as fast as I could. Finishing dinner Rick asked if I wanted some gum, it was blueberry Gum. My teeth blue and aching from the amount of sugar in it, it began to taste awful very quickly, spitting it out I asked if I could go for a smoke, the nurse at the counter says to me with a smile, you can go to the courtyard from the lounge Ben were just finishing the paper work so you can move to the front of the ward in the morning" "you can also relax in the lounge if you like but be back before nine p.m." walking past the security guard, I was growing anxious at how loud the ward sounded as I walked to the nurses' station. It was as though the aura of the ward felt like someone had died. I walk into the lounge and it was crowded. Little did I know that lot of the people here were suicide attempts over the holidays, they say that during Christmas is the worst time for mental illness cases. I found an empty seat near the radio of the lounge and walking to it I seen on the coffee table a pamphlet that had the word in bold SCHIZOPHRENIA the picture of it was an outline of a side profile of a person's head and it was outlined in barbed wire. Thinking my brain was surrounded by barbed wire around the halo I had visions of me on the cross next to Jesus with our crowns of thorn. Bleeding from the soul I flipped through the green covered pamphlet. Very dry mostly in medical terms it was describing what schizophrenia was and how it affected people clinically. Drowning in sorrow I feared this was going to be a lifelong fate for me, that my mind was now a prison and the unbearable thought of my own mortality I felt a loss that I will never be human again. Whispering to me was the music of Sandra, hearing it coming from my soul I listened and as if a dream of divine connection overcame me I realized she was on the radio again. I could never really understand why I had such a connection with a particular singer, but the words and melodies of the music entranced me to my core, I felt as though the songs were being prophesied. Thinking of how I wasted my life losing my opportunities with the fire department, breaking up with my old girlfriend Rachael Bowers. I was left asking myself why I am here on this earth. Even though in darkness I was terrified of dyeing I couldn't bear the thought of suicide, I felt as though there would be some higher purpose to my life, not knowing when or what would take place in my life I felt a calling of some sort, as though I was being called upon by god. My mind was so scrambled my entire religious belief was obliterated and I felt a loss for what this world thinks in laymen terms of iconic bible thumping Jesus. Nauseated I curled up on the sofa and wondered if I could predict the next time I would hear Sandra singing again, replaying that idea over and over I felt comfort in the psych ward as I rocked back and forth closing my eyes in a noise of peoples voices washing over me. Voices came over me while I sat in the lounge, voices of tragedy. "You should kill yourself" one would say, "You are nothing more than damnation!" "how do you expect to go on, everyone knows" being betrayed by my own thoughts was not something I could easily deal with, but something kept me here, something kept me existing in this life, I dreamt I had an ethereal child, a daughter, she was bright as a star shining between the earth and the moon, a beckon of light the world would see and follow to the end of time. In a place of hopelessness I raged to myself that I would not give up! This would not be my end, inwardly dyeing, I grasped desperately at anything I could to cope with my mental anguish. Rolling over in my bed and giving up was not going to happen, my family would have to dig my grave and bury me like a rabid dog in the wilderness before I would come to my demise. In waves I'd feel anxiety of damnation and trying to counter that I tried to think of what it would be like to be a friend of Sandra's even though I was just a stranger lost in a strange place, what kind of life would it take to just ask, will you be my friend Sandra? I felt ashamed of myself so much that such a question would be absurd. I was not worthy of even my own mind.

## Chapter 3

My uncle told me he was going flying for the day. I said ok and put on my headset and started to draw in my sketchbook. No sooner did he leave my heart thumped so hard it jolted me and with a ringing in my ears I heard my name loud like a trumpet "Ben!" thinking it was my uncle giving me hell I took off my headset and started to look around his basement suite. There was no one there, the TV was off and it was quite. I began to dwell on the voice I thought I shouldn't be here; god is trying to tell me to go to the waterfront. I hopped in the shower and took off in my car to the bus stop. When I arrived at the bus stop, it was sunny out. I slipped on the ice at the curb; the fall weather was getting chilly. I looked up in the sky and the moon was shining through the blue sky. I stood there for quite some time seeing several busses but not the 401 bus. I began to feel rage and thought I should start walking to make a path. I stepped on the grass and dragged my feet walking faster and faster in a perfect circle. Soon people began to ask what I was doing the more they asked the more I contorted my body and started to breath really heavy. Several hours had passed the moon began to sink closer to the horizon. Someone got off one of the busses and walked in my area where I was walking. He completely ignored what I was doing and I wanted to beat the crap out of him. It took all my will not to do anything. I kept walking and a single mom started showing her three year old daughter my engraving in the grass. The only person who was complimenting me on what I was doing. Thinking to myself I began to imagining that the TV people would come and start filming me I was going to be famous, they would see me walking in this circle and I would bring everyone on earth to their knees as I flew off the earth around the buildings and past the moon. Time passed and soon a RCMP car

43

pulls to the curb, a man and woman RCMP member come to see what I was doing. All the sudden the woman cop tries to forcibly subdue me. I wiggle out of her grasp and she started to yell "did you see him hit me!!" The male officer pulled out a can of pepper spray and sprayed my eyes. Not feeling the effects for several minutes the officers became very worried. Then the mace hit my eyes, burning my forehead. I lost my footing and fell to the ground. I split my brow when I hit the phone booth at bus stop. The officers were on me faster than lighting, but there were now six of them. I just went limp and let them cuff me. An officer shouted he can walk into the ambulance, they tried to stand me up but I played as if I was unconscious. Tossing me in the ambulance an officer said in astonishment "he burned a path in the ground." as I was laying in the ambulance the attendant inside started to drill me. "You better tell me what's wrong with you" "you're going to the hospital and if you don't tell me the doctors are going to fill you with drugs are that what you want?" I still made out like I was unconscious and let the dick bag ramble. Thinking to myself yes you fill me with your poisons I will adapt and destroy all of you. They wheeled me into emergency and I clutched the steel on the frame of the bed and locked up my body. They tried to roll me over to stitch my forehead. An officer told the attending doctor that I couldn't be rolled over I was like a vice. After I lay with my face in the pillow I decided to let them work on me. I rolled over the cuffs dug right into my wrists and I chirped in pain. Telling the doctor to take these fucking cuffs off me, he said in a rather harsh voice, "Sorry son those cuffs stay on till I am done working on you!" Trying to roll so they wouldn't feel like they were cutting my hands off I squirmed to no relief. The more I moved the more the cuffs dug in. after the doctor stitched me up, they took the cuffs off and I ask for some water. I had an uncontrollable thirst. They gave me these little paper cups; I must have asked the nurse to get me water ten times. I became more aware of where I was they lead me to a room that had no windows. It was made of cinder blocks and there was a small mattress in the room. I lay down and was asleep instantly. I awoke to a click of a pen, "hello" a nurse said "I am from mental health" unable to keep my eyes open and slipping in and out of consciousness she said to me " I would like to ask you some questions" I tried to fight the urge to sleep with all my might and I muttered the word "ok." She talked, asking me if I was on any drugs, I said no but I did smoke a joint the previous night. Then she said "well do you know that cannabis can trigger chemical imbalances in the brain?" trying to answer I said "no." then I kept hearing a beeping, the nurse apologizing for her pager constantly going off. I couldn't fight the urge to sleep anymore and was unconscious again. I awoke later to the sound of my aunt's voice. "Ben" she whispered, I murmured a response. She asked "why did I go and do that? Did you know your uncle found your car with the keys on the seat of your car?" I was trying to tell her something but no words were coming out of my mouth. I felt like giving up. My aunt then tells me that the officers would like to apologize for their treatment of you, I said "ok." They walked in and started to joke with me asking if I was part of a rugby team. Concerned they told my aunt there was a bad case of mushrooms on the streets and worried I might have taken some. To their relief I didn't take any. Before the released me I had to talk to a psychiatrist. I walked into the office still barley able to keep my eyes open; I was asked several difficult questions. The one that sticks in my mind were he said "do you believe in any religions?" I told him I believe in all religions, thinking to myself I will be waiting for you when the time comes. After a few more questions that I really couldn't answer due to the fact I felt like my mind as being put threw a blender. The doctor put me back in the custody of my uncle and aunt. My uncle calling me space man the whole night and I was so ashamed at what I did I just wanted to go to bed completely exhausted from the whole ordeal. The Flashback of that memory was almost too much to bear as I sat waiting for my mom in the lounge of the psych ward. My uncle told me after that, the doctor said it was a psychotic breakdown, and that I was a very disturbed individual. I wasn't too pleased when I heard that from my uncle, and thought what the fuck does a doctor know seeing me half unconscious for fifteen minutes? Later some explanations would be I was having a spiritual awakening, thinking about this it did feel very spiritual but it terrified me to the very core of my being. My brain was on fire as I sat on the sofa on the lounge, people talking in rolling waves there was no piece and quite in the psych ward of One South tonight. Doctor Alan told me in an appointment it is unusual for people to remember there psychotic episodes, but for me I had a detailed photographic memory of what happened. Nauseous overcoming me all I wanted was silence in my head and in the lounge. The voices of people talking coupled with the voices I was listening to in my mind was making it like there would be no way out for peace and quiet. Walking in the psych ward Alice and Steve went to the nurses counter, astonished at how busy the ward was they asked where I was, a nurse replying " Ben is in the lounge" walking into the lounge my mom took one look at me and asked if I was ok? Looking at her half sedated I replied no I can't stand it here. Alice told Steve to ask a nurse if there was somewhere quiet we could go to. Steve came back and taking Alice and myself showing us to a TV room. "Ben the nurse said if you need some peace and quiet you can come here into the TV room." the room small and dank and smelled moldy from the ninety seventies furniture it wasn't a big room but at least I could find some solitude while the psych ward was how could I say being insane over the holidays! My mom reaching into her purse says to me " Look what we brought for you Ben" pulling out one of my black tattered sketchbooks I had while I was attending Vancouver animation school, I looked as though I was being saved from my mental chaos. While attending the Vancouver animation school the only outlet I had to express myself was writing in my sketchbook accompanied by drawing minute images of what the world looked like to me and how the angels of my damnation hunted me. My mom handed me a small case of pens and pencils and smiling she said "I knew you would like this" worried that if they looked at it, it would incriminate me in some way writing psychotic thoughts in the book, but Alice explained to me that doctor Alan read what I wrote and there was nothing to worry about I wouldn't go to jail for writing what was in there. What I was trying to do was write about a love story between humanity and living in heaven among the angels, but what really went from pen to paper was me challenging a demon with words of hate and anguish. Filling a demon with hate and challenging him, I later found out is not the best thing to do. In reflecting back to what I wrote I guess the damnation I felt was the after effects of being thwarted by darkness and my longing for redemption was indeed a true feeling of something I had to do. Soon one of the older women that I recognized from the shed who butted out Jesus came in the room to watch TV. Uncomfortable I began to squirm with inpatients of how she could disturb me and my family. Alice assuring me its ok, she tried to calm me down. Looking through the blinds of the window of the room I could see it was dark and the lights of the hospital and city were comforting. Crying to my mom I don't want to stay here people here are crazy. Sympathizing my mom explained that I'll have to stay here for a while till my meds stabilize my chemical imbalance. The feeling of losing control was above excruciating. Soon Steve's biological father the man who raised me but was my step father Wayne came to see me. He sat with me trying to comfort me, I never really agreed with him while growing up. A lot of the time we fought because I just wanted to be a care free kid growing up and he always wanted me to be a hard worker, but the reality was even in my school work I couldn't be academic or bust my ass so to speak. However during my short time before I was in high school and the time I went to Vancouver animation school I had my share of back breaking jobs most of them worth more than the minimum wage I earned from them. During high school I graduated with mostly art credits my forte was being an artist, I also had a way with philosophy and used it as a way to express my creativity. When I graduated I was nineteen, able to get into the nightclubs and bars yet unable to be seen as an adult while in high school. My mother and Wayne remained friends after they divorced and even though my mom remarried Wayne was able to find his own path in life. I still called Wayne dad and happy to see him he was telling me he wanted me to come for dinner after I get out of the hospital to meet his new girlfriend. Excited for him I said ok, he went on to tell me she is an artist and I would like her. Her name was Pam and she planned on cooking a roast for dinner when I was out of the hospital. My family sat with me until it was time for bed, I wandered back to the end of one south and waving goodbye to my family went in my room closed the door and slipped under the covers of the hospital bed. Waking up the breakfast cart was about to pack up leavening me a plateful, this time it was porridge and dry toast with some tasteless strawberries. I think that day it was easier to choke down my medication then it was for me to eat the hospital food. The nurse told me to take my belongings they had a room for me ready. When I went to my new room I was sharing it with and elderly person the nurse told me not to worry about him he doesn't leave his room. When entering the room all I could see of him was that he was wearing jeans and dress socks. The nurse leaving me handed me my packs of cigarettes explaining that I could smoke them as much as I wanted but to make sure I hid them very well patients come into the room's and steel them. I looked at the night stand next to my bed shoving my belongings inside I burred my smokes as best I could and took my sketch book and one of my mechanical pen's and decide to sit in the lounge. The psych ward seemed like it was completely different there wasn't nearly as much activity, later I found out a lot of people were discharged and even more were on day passes to go home. Walking into the lounge I seen that a janitor was disassembling the Christmas tree, there was a few people sitting in the lounge some were on the sofas reading others were at the tables finishing breakfast, and as I looked around I seen that the chair next to the radio was open. I sat down and closing my eyes I began to write. The writing was mostly nonsense just me having discussions with myself. Or rather having discussions with what the voices were saying in my mind. Even though I felt in prison in my mind when I was writing I felt I could write without boundaries or limitations. The writing flowed almost as fluent as drawing a picture. Feeling a freedom I let my pen cover pages of the sketchbook. If I were to put the words into context it would be like the writing of a very underdeveloped teenager who didn't pass grade eleven special needs course. Never the less I wrote and I dreamed that one day I will write a novel about my life experience in the psych ward of One South. The task almost seemed daunting I thought I would be famous that the riches of my writing would forever be known as an award winning novel. Laughing at this, it was the only glimpse of joy I thought about, I now had a new purpose to my life to somehow bring my experiences to people that not only were ill but also who lived with family members of such a crippling illness. But in cold reality I was nowhere near skilled nor in the right mind frame to make anything did I write legible. Hours past and I was writing and drawing occasionally I would hear Sandra singing imagining I was locked in a castle that the demon I was facing was a monster. In a moment of clarity I wrote "A Cold voice whispers to me. "It's true!" On the wings of an owl I flutter. Through the night's trees, the stars still with shadows of the trees rushing by. Dew drops fall to the forest floor from the Breeze of the crisp night's air. I am locked in a little room in this tree. I gaze at the moon so full and perfect through the rooms only window. My senses on fire, oh how I do love her so! She is with me in this room. We are children who disobeyed. Bound together in our hearts we sit on our pedestals like trophies of an age forgotten. However this came to be we just know it's true forever. Her Name is Sandra, Butterflies and places where coconuts grow, her name sinks in my heart. Something though made me get off my pedestal. A feeling of doom a feeling I was not meant to stay in this prison as a trophy. Unstoppable are the tears flowing from my unborn jaw. I feel an overwhelming sorrow. I look back at Sandra and I did once feel innocence in her presence. But the time has come. I step on the window sill looking down at the earth. I fall from the highest branch of the looming tree. A baby Cry's a new life. Born unto earth my wings flutter. Glowing my heart thumps and soon Angels kiss my forehead and I feel it tickle inside my mind. My ears begin to ring softly singing". And in writing these words I felt as though I was possessed, angry at myself for making this person who I never met, into something that was not true. I began damning myself for being sensitive to emotions. I tore the pedestal I held her on and fought the obsession, however it seemed in my mind of a calling of angels to my soul. Tormented and weak I knew that this illusion I was placing was nothing more than an irrational thought. Haunting me as I sat and wrote in my sketchbook I raged against myself for feeling something other than death. Muttering to myself I whispered 'to feel pure joy and happiness is to die again and again and again. I wrote "I drop my cross and lose my way, I fly by night again and again and again." trying to cope I began my rocking in my chair. The day continued on and a nurse who was in street clothing came up to me. "Hello Ben my name is Cindy, I hold the life skills program during the weekdays, would you like to join us tomorrow?" nodding my head I said ok, smiling she says "Great I'll see you tomorrow at ten am" feeling like I had no choice now but to attend, a feeling of anxiety and panic washed over me like storming rain over wilted flowers. Every moment was inspiration for my little black sketchbook and every moment was in the same context damnation. "The Medications are different." I wrote, considering the fact it was probably smoking cannabis from the age of fifteen to now the age of twenty two that contributed to my psychosis. Ironically I was being placed on more drugs called anti psychotics to become stable and soon leave the hospital. The idea of fighting drugs with drugs was almost the same idea as fighting the devil with the devil. I began to write. "Dancing in the twilight of dawns sky I was the morning star , shaking my fists at god, I was in damnation of existence, how much courage would it take to be the ONLY ONE" in an instance I flashed back to the cold road of the Coquihalla. Floating in and out of consciousness I see the headlights of an oncoming car, lights going from one light to two lights back to one. Thinking this was code for my upcoming death my mind wandered to when I was only a baby. I remember seeing lights in the sky and thinking of a blimp in the night's sky. I was thinking this,  seeing the hand of my friends girlfriend slap a note to my forehead, "Stick that in your pipe and smoke it!" she said, drifting I see images of god walking in gold pastures of wheat wearing a white suit. "You will be with me soon my son." Drifting and looking at the stars threw the trees. Bright they were twinkling I imagined them as angels on pedestals. At that moment I seen one fall to earth. Eyes wide open looking out the window I seen angels hunting me. They cut across the cold forest floor as swift as I can think of them. Slicing my head with swords they cross the road I catch a glimpse of them returning to their pedestals and I hear a voice say "that was easy!" sorrow fills my heart then rage. I say out loud "I am coming for you!" "Oh yes they will pay". Seeing lights in the distance I am eager to use a washroom. The man in the car stating we were almost there. We stop at a local filling station and I use the restroom. I return outside and the man says "sorry friend this is as far as you go." I look around no clue where I am I see down the road a twenty four hour corner store. They leave the station and I begin to walk. I arrive to the store and decide I should get a pop to drink. I buy it and head over to the magazines. I begin to absorbed all the magazines and think of the powers I attained from the video game ones. I walked back and forth around the store I would place my pop on the floor and find it in different parts of the store. A lady then says to me "sir you can't stay here." not knowing where to go, I head across the road to a low budget strip mall. I walked up to the bench and seen the yellow curb paint go in a half circle. My mind raced and I vision an asteroid would come to wipe out the earth only we would be saved by divine intervention. I see the mind of god and the body of god. A two dimensional being trapped in a cold eternity of a tomb and the only way to let the light in is by sending souls to live in the universe as nerves of light slowly breaking away the cold darkness. I look up at the moon cursing under my breath. I see a shadow as if a person was walking across the moon leaving her shadow to be seen from earth. I wake from my little visions and walk across the road back to the corner store. Barely able to keep myself up I stand there my legs nearly buckling under my weight. I walk to the teller and ask to buy several packs of cigarettes. I didn't have any money but I did have a charge card. When she handed me the slip to sign my name I started to cry. Thinking to myself I am about to sign my life away for what? Cigarettes, in my mind I see Sandra looking at me threw the stores windows holding a child scowling and cursing me for doing such a thing. I cry, mad at myself I sign my name and scratch it out several times. The teller concerned frequently asking me if I am alright. I weep and nod. I leave the store with my smokes constantly lighting them and instantly flicking them on the ground. The cigarettes tasted like waste from a toxic dump. I go to walk back in the store and a RCMP officer stops me. "Sir Can I have your ID please?" the officer asks. I hand him my driver's license. "Did your family report you missing sir?" not knowing the answer to the question I stated a low mutter "yes?" I am going to take you to the station sir please step into the car. I sit in the seat and close my eyes, awaking instantly to the cars chirp and flash of red and blue. Rocking in the psych wards lounge chair I write in my sketchbook, "You are the damnation and you will never find me!" "I Fly By Night Again!" and again I die inside like a falling star losing its light in the nights sky. The memory I had did not sit well in my stomach. With a crash I hear the lunch cart come through the front lobby doors, it stops in the lounge and people begin to take their lunch. I walk over to the cart and took a tray; the hospital food is becoming less appetizing as I find that the cooking seems to have lost its lustre. This would be my routine for the next few weeks, sitting in the chair writing and drawing listening to the radio eventually my medications would get changed till I was on two milligrams of Risperdal, and I would continue to show improvements while in the psych ward. I did attend the daily life skills program with Cindy while in the psych ward but making ashtrays out of chipped tiles and grout was not my idea of therapy. Something interesting did occur during my sessions in the life skills program, I already knew that Edgar Alan Poe was a schizophrenic but I did not realize that so was Winston Churchill, and Howard Hues. There was something in those people, a bit of inspiration to continue moving forward in my life. One South was not a fun place to be, the building itself was separate from the Kamloops hospital almost like we were not part of the medical community. Segregating filled the mental health of peoples recovery , I found it very unreasonable that in reality cancer although a very serious illness received the most of the entire medical funding while building resort like hospitals for people with cancer, people with other illnesses were left with very little funding. The psychiatric community couldn't figure out why people with a mental illness never seemed to recover, my question to that is being medicated to sedation and locked on a single bed room with one caged window was supposed to inspire someone to recover? Later I would find out that the schizophrenic society of Kamloops received little if any funding for support after leavening the psych ward and try to begin to sort out my life I was left with little to no support other than my family. It was going to be up to me to decide if I just roll over in my bed and give up or try to live somewhat normal life. Still unable to trust myself I was able to come home. I lay in bed wondering what will come of me, hearing the children in the day-care I thought if only I was that age again able to start over and know everything I know now. Still having a bit of hallucinations and hearing dreadful voices. I needed to find something to make my life have meaning something to give me inspiration to not give up, being told by my psychiatrist doctor Alan, that I probably would not be able to get a job or go to school, and being only twenty two, It seemed I would be having a lot of time on my hands to dwell and mull in the devices of my own mind. I was going to be discovering that while being a man a lot of people would think in society I was nothing without some sort of monetary income or not a man if I couldn't work. It's funny what we grow up into with the dogmatic vision society holds towards people. Waiting for the sky to fall and wondering what could I possibly do now that I had all the time in the world I had an appointment with Doctor Alan to discuss my disability pension? This would of course be my only means of support from society and it wasn't a get rich kind of support in fact it's far below the poverty line that Canada's government considers, which without  question the amount I received would in fact have put me on the streets if I did not have a family to help support me. Pulling out of the driveway from my home in Rayleigh, I put in one of Sandra's CD's into my cars stereo. It was five P.M. already dark outside and I was headed to Wayne's apartment for a roast dinner. Alice reminding me to drive very carefully while going to Wayne's the roads are slippery this time of year. My mind still fogged with visions of me being on an epic prophecy to bring heaven to earth. I was showing signs of become balanced every day, yet the images in my mind were still strong. It was only a few weeks after being released from One South, but from the meds they weight gain was extremely fast already having quite the pot belly all along my waistline was stretch marks of the rapid weight gain. Driving south along the freeway I could see above the horizon line of the mountains a bright star fallowing me. Like a beacon of truth with Sandra singing her music it was almost surreal of lost time. The melodies washing over me like an angel whispers to a mortals soul, I felt entranced by the evening. Watching the lights of the city become more prominent, I approached the town. I felt a sense of piece driving in the cold winter's night. I arrived at Wayne's apartment unscathed, wondering what his new girlfriend was like I was interested in what kind of artist she was., I knocked on the door and Pam greeted me with a hug introducing herself she had taken my jacket and I took off my shoes. Seeing she was a painter I asked what medium she used, she replied she panted with acrylics. She pointed to a small picture on the wall abstract she asked me "do you know what this is Ben?" I looked at the panting and said " There Eyes" laughing she said " See Wayne Ben knows what this painting is." she began to tell me that while I went missing Wayne was in bed and then out of nowhere they were surrounded by eyes. Not too sure what she was talking about and envisioning this while still having glimpses of my psychosis it only affirmed to me that something great had happened when I went missing. Pam asked me if I would like to paint something we had a bit of time before the roast would be done, I said ok, wondering if she had a spare canvas. Walking into the living room I seen her easel in the corner next to the dining room table, and leaning next to it was framed wood and a roll of sheeted canvas. We're going to build our own canvas Ben how big would you like to make it? Picking the size of a smaller sized canvas she built it within five minutes and primed it then sat it on her easel and let me mix my paints. Painting the picture wasn't anything in particular I mostly wanted to capture a mood rather than an actual tangible object. She began laughing and muttering to herself, wondering why she was sort of talking to someone who wasn't there she later explained to me she was talking to her spirit guides who she could see. I myself was always fascinated with psychic phenomena, but never really understood it, the night progressed and while eating dinner, she would be off talking to her guides and Wayne and I quietly ate our dinner. The night seemed very unusual and I began to wonder am I really in this world or just a figment of my own imagination. After finishing dinner and spending time with Wayne and the Empathic I left saying my goodbyes and started my car and began to drive home, while I drove listening to Sandra I had a flashback to when I was entering my psychotic breakdown.

Cory Kaldal

## Chapter 4

My heart and mind were open now. Like a flood of love coming in, I had a vision after working a graveyard shift at the gas station I worked at. The more I hated myself, the more I criticized and the smaller I made myself in my mind. The more I felt euphoric and in love with everything around me. I began in my mind to take who I was and tear it down bit by bit till one day I no longer existed in my mind. Little did I know this was leading me to a state of mind that I could never come back from? I was opening a door that could never be closed. I started down this path, there was no looking back to the person I once was. I lie down in my bed after work and put on a CD of a female artist that I was not too sure of. I listened to her voice and began to lift into the air floating off my bed. Off the earth, out of my realm of reality, I floated past my life, past time and space, till I was no longer at home, but in the presence of the almighty. I basked in the presence of love, my mind's eye on fire my heart open. After a few minutes a fear came over me. What if I am dead? My heart nearly went through my chest and I began to fall back down to my bed. Fear stabbing my heart like a cold knife. I felt out of place. My mind silenced and I could not speak. I later fell asleep but now I was beyond anyone's help. I thought this was who I am, this is what I will be and I am going to show everyone how to do it! Thinking how foolish this vision was and how I could be so misled by my thoughts I went on in condemning myself of my psychotic breakdown and began to remember more. I felt a calling to what I was about to do, this would change my life and everyone else's lives as well. The vision I had was still fresh in my mind with the feeling of my soul on fire. I began to obsess about religion. I felt the more books on new age and spiritual books, the bible, the more I would become a part of god. I felt myself no longer a man but an angel of god. One who would take the earth and bring heaven unto it. I felt as though I would ascend to heaven and am the one to cross the threshold from the living to the dead. The way I would do this was by what I manifested during the day. The more I had things take place in my life the more I would be lead to the path to god. I started to read everything I could get my hands on. Every word began to resonate with me whether it is the newspaper or comic books. Slowly I began to cross from what was real to what were just words on paper. Then something strange happened to me, I noticed I could absorb things that people told me, things that I heard around me. Things I seen, everything that I lived was a beginning in a new world. I was on my last few graveyard shifts at work before I was going to school and I happened to notice someone left a kung Fu book at work. I read it and I became aware that I could do anything from kung Fu. I decided I needed to practice but only the way I knew how. I began to walk on tipsy toes and jump up and down while I was at work. I would ring in people's purchases as fast and as loud as I could on the till. Every word I read was making sense and pointing me to a higher existence. It all was code for me to decipher. I felt I could learn how to do anything and whatever I absorbed made me a stronger angel of god. I was still longing for companionship though. I was eager to move to my uncles because the city was waiting for me. I knew I would find my destiny there._The time for me to move to my uncles has come. I spent a few days packing my things. Cloths, sketchbooks, music, and my car were loaded to the brim. I drove off, my parents waving bye. I felt that I was starting down a path that would change the way people look at life. The world was an organism shaped by one spiritual being. The air was crisp that day and with the sun dancing in and out of the clouds I drove as fast as I could. I rolled down the window. My car bounced down the freeway, bottoming out on the ruts in the road left by the truck drivers. Two eagles in the sky circling over the tree tops of the freeway. I watched them and I could see tracers float off their wing tips. They are angles I thought to myself, floating to see me off to the way to god. Even though I was speeding there were cars passing me in a whispering sound? I could see tracers and auras of the cars passing bye. I thought I was becoming more in tune with the spiritual realm. I drove to the lower mainland noticing that most people were driving beaters. They were passing me like maniacs. I thought to myself how people are in such a rush to get to places they know nothing of. They are all lost sheep trying to find where I was going. They all know what will happen. It won't be pleasant. I will be the first and the last and I will bring you all with me. My mind floats with the world at its end. Nature began taking its root over time. We all will live to see it after it's all gone. Then what? Who will be in charge that will see that we must live among the earth and heaven as one? I see the storm clouds approach the earth and people being washed away by the sea, helpless people drowning in their own sorrow. The eternity of it all so bleak I wonder if there is hope for us. Getting closer to my uncles I notice a car pass me with a cross hanging in a rear view mirror. Seeing huge tracers from the cross I think to myself he is burning his soul in hell. The memories of the past sicken me I begin to think I am nothing more than a bunch of lies. Feeling sick to my stomach and the weight of anxiety washing over me, I pull into my homes driveway exhausted coming from Wayne's apartment. I walk in the door and head to my bedroom ready to crash for the night, sleeping I have more nightmares of leaving my body. I awake Groggy and in a stupor, the drugs taking their toll making me more lethargic each day that passes. Doctor Alan said one of the side effects with Risperdal would be rigidity in the muscles, feeling like I've been dragged through the mud I wander into the kitchen and make myself some coffee. Alice reminded me I had a doctor's appointment with doctor Alan this morning, I began to get dressed and prepare myself for the task of speaking to the doctor. Sitting in the doctor's office I flip through a magazine, wanting to get the appointment over and done with we finally get called into Doctor Alan's office. Alice had been taking great pains to observe my behavior and I began to tell the doctor of the nightmares I was continuing having. He prescribes another experimental drug called Celexa and ups the dose of my Risperdal to three milligrams. After taking several notes into my medical record we then leave the office and reschedule another appointment. Alice and I get in the car and head over to the Grocery Store to fill our prescriptions. Driving across town I start remembering parts of my psychotic breakdown. We eat dinner that night and I try for an early bed time. My uncle is working in the morning and I wanted to get my route to the school a go through, because it is a very long commute. They watch the evening news, and I find a place on the living room floor and begin to contort my body in a fashion that leaves my aunt and uncle pondering what I am doing. After I do my contortions I tell them I am off to bed and watching the news I know they can tell what I am thinking. I wake up early, have a shower and get dressed to start the practice run to school it's a Saturday. Listening to my music and with my prophecy books in hand I feel I will see her today. My heart is filled with sorrow as I drive to the bus stop where I will head to the sky train station. I get on the bus. I needed to memorize the number it was the 401 bus. I had a seat to myself and my music thumping probably too loud, people were defiantly staring at me. The bus drives off down the freeway I notice it's a rather warm day and I had a pretty heavy coat on, the sun coming through the tinted window. Beads of sweat were rolling from my brow. I get off the bus and walk up the stations escalators deciding to run up them dodging the people standing on them. I run up noticing out of the corner of my eye a girl smiling running down the stairs next to the escalator. I start to laugh thinking perfect what else can I manifest for the day. Getting onto the sky train I hear voices in conversation talking to faint to understand what they're saying yet load enough to know it's a man and women. I look around and see no one engaged in conversation everyone just taking their seats. I sit next to the window and watch the city whisk by the train. Beads of sweat still rolling off my brow I stretch out my hands and contort them so there fully extended fingertip to fingertip. A bead of sweat begins to form at my index fingertips. I ponder if the sun is touching my finger and boiling my blood. My soul feels like it's on fire and my ears are burning with noise. I hear the intercom say "Cross Roads" and decide to exit the train. I will find her around the corner I thought. I walk the city street seeing people pass by laughing, I had my pack with me filled with sketchbooks art supplies, and my prophecy books. I listen to my favorite singer and look up at the condos that stretch into the sky. I see there auras go past the buildings into the sky as far as the eye can see. I truly felt like the architect of god. I wander the streets; the road comes to another train station. I begin to laugh! See how you lead me? Thank you for bringing me back to where I need to go! I get back onto the train and continue my trek to the school. I get off at the last destination of the train. The waterfront! I run up the stations long causeway to the main lobby of the station. I walk into the station and gasp. There are murals on the ceiling of angels and cherubs carved into the stone of the building; the whole architecture of the building takes my breath away. I walk outside to see a statue of arch angel Michel leading a lost soul to heaven. In awe I know that where I go from here is very much a part of my destiny. I decide to walk along the waterfronts stores and café's watching the people hustle and bustle to where ever they tend to go in such a hurry. I decide to have a coffee at the stars. I order my usual hot frothy beverage and find a place outside to take it all in. I sit and start to shoot people with my mind's eye, tagging them. Who will be worthy of my thinking and who will be led astray. I sit laughing to myself oh this will be the way for others to come. I gaze up looking at the city's sky line to notice that there are three rings around the towers peak. "The father, son and holy ghost" I giggled. Sitting at the cafe I began to hear voices over my headset. Not knowing who they were I took my headset off and heard just traffic of the cars flying down the city streets. Not thinking anything of it I put my headset back on, finished my coffee and decided to start to wander the streets. Seeing if I could find any sign of the women who would be my destiny. I walked along the streets; I was looking in windows of shops thinking what part of her I would find and where I would meet her. All this made me search even more diligently. I smiled as I walked and all the sudden I heard a voice say in my mind " I hate leather!" taking off my headset I didn't hear anything again but the sound of cars roaring down the city streets, taxies honking at the lights. I walk down more city blocks and come across a mall under the ground. I go into the mall and start browsing the shops absorbing everything there is in the shops windows. Picking out the things she likes and destroying things she doesn't all of it so funny I can hardly stand it. With a POP the strap I was holding my pack with blew the stitch and the pack fell to the ground with a thud. I thought ha-ha one's own thoughts are heavy how funny. I take the other strap and keep walking with one strap dangling from the other end. I keep walking around the mall and I find myself heading to the sky train station, walking down escalators. I thought how convenient I guess it's time to go home. With that thought I was on the train to see it was already dark out with the city lights aglow. I would dwell on these thoughts for ten years I began to think of the rest of what happened before my parents found me remembering the events my eyes glaze over and I begin to envision the events that followed. I drove to the bus stop all I could think about was if someone would recognize me from the day before walking in a circle. I parked my car and headed for the bus as it was already there. I quickly got on and tried to find a window seat. The bus was overly crowded as most people were heading to work or school on it. We got to the station where I caught the sky train and the place was packed like a zoo. Was very busy today, morning rush had started and everyone's day was about to begin. I was timing myself, I thought wow this is a very long commute. By the time I hit the waterfront it was a total of 3 hours from my uncles just one way. So I walked the streets of the waterfront I decided to have a coffee under the stars and try and still wake up when I got to the coffee shop it was 7:30 am. The school when it started was scheduled to open at 8 am. Which made every day a very long day seeing as it was 3 hours just to get there. School was over at 5pm and usually we did homework there because the courses were cram courses and then 3 hours home. The school was all about cramming as much as they could into one years' worth of curriculum; it was basically 4 years of work crammed into one year. I sat under the stars sipping my coffee and watching the sun slowly creep into the morning sky I began to think that the end will be soon for all of us. Today I will find the cloths she will love. Thinking for a while of what her name was and then it came to me, her name is Sandra. I went back into the café and sat at my table, I pulled off the black leather gloves I was wearing and thought these hands are not mine they are "his" I must discard them. I left my gloves at the table and quickly walked out of the café.

Disposing of my coffee cup I decided to find the things Sandra wanted. I thought to myself where would an angel go to give her gifts and where in the city would we live? Of course an angel of god would only live in a luxury suite. I would fly from the roof tops into the green night's sky having my wife cooking dinner. This would be my portal to other dimensions I would be observing life on different plains of existence. Now where would an angel live? Slowly I wandered the streets until I came to hotel Vancouver. I walked inside the posh establishment and began to browse its fine architecture. While I was wandering inside I thought ah we would be in the penthouse, so I found the closest elevator and hit the very top button on the consol. There was a few people getting off at different floors but as the last one got off I went to the very top floor in the elevator alone. When I stepped onto the floor at the top I felt a bit dizzy looking out of the windows I was pretty high up. Walking like I was on a balance beam I went to the end of the hall and knocked on the door. Of course I expected Sandra to be there opening the door with open arms hugging and kissing me. She would be dressed in white jeans and a very comfortable sweater I thought. With a whoosh a side door opened and a maid came out of the room. "Oh I am sorry sir there is no one in the suite today." Oh! I replied, thanks for the info. I walked cautiously back to the elevator and down to the lobby. When I went down to the lobby my ears began to pop here and there. Disappointed she wasn't home I left the hotel threw the huge double doors pushing them so hard they slammed against the walls. I walked along the street I came across the cities music store. It had every kind of music, video game, and comic books I could ever dream of. I walked through the store looking for the right kind of music she would like. I came to one artist and started to stare at the cover. Then all the sudden POP, the other strap to my pack blew out and my pack hit the ground with a thud!

Thinking the weight of god's work is extremely heavy I clasped my pack by the hook strap and now I had two straps dangling. This pack is getting more awkward to carry daily. I end up heading towards the comic book section of the store. Gaining all the powers of the super heroes I had seen. I come across a comic about a boy who could travel to different dimensions, fascinated I buy the comic and head over to the stores bistro. Reading over the comic I realize its telling my life story and these are the places I will be going to once I have ascended. It was as if it was a map to where I was destined to go like my story was foretold as a prophecy. I ate lunch and began to smile knowing what I had to do now. I left running through the store and jumping on the sidewalk out the doors. I slap my hands together and rub them furiously and in a small voice I say to myself "Excellent!" now moving faster I come to the underground mall and remembered I needed to get cloths for school I open the door and run inside. I browse the shops and boutiques for things Sandra would love to have. I come across a video store and on a green poster I see the title V. thinking to myself ah, Roman numeral number five. I purchase the video set and put it in my already overburdened pack. My aunt Shirley will love these. I was thinking of an early Christmas present. I walk through the mall and not finding any cloths I liked, I thought maybe I would like a few dress shirts. I walk into a suit store for men and start to look at the cloths. A man comes up to me and says are you looking for a suit today sir? I say I am not too sure I am mostly looking at shirts. He says well how bout we try some of these jackets on. I take a look at a few and try some on. He says I know this one would be perfect! I thought my uncle would love a suit maybe we could hit the town some night all dressed up. The man asked me "will you be getting pants today too sir?" what do they look like I asked. He says I know which ones would be perfect with that jacket. Of course he comes back with a tie and shirt as well. I get everything on and thought I looked really good. Shall I put them in a bag for you sir? Ok I said. After he finishes ringing in the total he says to me "that will be $475 dollars" I tell him I can't afford that it's my whole months budget! Yes sir but these are on sale now; you won't find better savings then this anywhere! I say to myself yes of course the savings I hand him my debit card and walk out of the store with my new cloths. Feeling awkward I wondered how I would afford more cloths. I walk around some more and then decide to head home after all I had a three hour ride to get home and it was already getting late. After I arrived home I showed my uncle and aunt my suit and puzzled they said to me " A suit?" then I told them with glee I thought me and Leland could hit the town one night. My uncle asked me how much it was, I told him. Very upset with me he said "Now what are you going to do for money?" I shrugged and said I don't know but I'll think of something. I decide I was going to take a nap I had a very long day and was bushed. I went in my room and cranked my music and my bedroom had a very strong scent of roses. I thought my body smells like roses because I am closer to god. I close my eyes and I could see all the angels of heaven lining up for me to start my ascension. With swords overhead and smoke coming from their eyes I begin to dance in my bed to my music. The smell of the sweet roses consumes me and I head for the light of god. I wake up during the night and begin to think I don't need my eyes to see, if I put my thumbs in my sockets I could see threw my fingers. This is how all angels see. I then try and stab my eyes with my thumbs hoping to gouge them out. The harder I push on my eyes the more I feel euphoric. Then I realize I cannot shatter the two things I love the most. I lay in bed, my toe begins to cramp and burn I extend my toe so it cramps even more and I think to myself my toe is standing on Jupiter and my mind reaches past the sun. Then I grasp the air around me clenching my hand to a fist and tugging. I can grasp my soul I know where it is. And I drift off to sleep. I awake to a very loud CLICK! The light turns on the desk. The hand of god has awoken me I thought. 30 minutes before my alarm would wake me up groggy I go have my shower and skip coffee and breakfast. I'll have coffee under the stars I thought. I get in my car and the puddles from the night's rain are frozen to the ground. I decide to take the freeway today and as I listen to the radio I hear Sandra singing. Astonished I turn it up. I am on my way I said to myself. I park the car at the bus stop, waiting for my bus. Today was our orientation day at school and we needed to get paper work done such as student loans and pictures taken for ID.I had my coffee under the stars and was staring at what I deemed the three kings. I noticed they put up lights on the tower that flashed different colors. Happy I thought yes those people know I am coming. I sit down and a man asks me for a smoke. I gladly give him one. Smiling he asks what I am listening too. I said Sandra. He smiles "yes she's one of my favorites too." Did you know she was live at the colossus music store? I go really?? He replies "yes" I thought to myself she is following me. The man walks off great full for the cigarette and looking back smiling. All I could do is staring as he walked off. Thinking ah ha a messenger of the coming tides. I start to walk to the school and see people gathering. I of course introduce myself to my new classmates and watch as different people start to line up outside the schools doors. When the school opens we are showed our classroom and then gather to be taken to do financing as well as get our photos for our ID. When we are getting our photos done someone commented that there are twelve men and only one woman. I thought these people will be my apostles and show other people where I go. We are sent to a theatre to go over the policies of the school and some very harsh rules. I of course know they don't apply to me. We leave the theatre, we are handed our ID and I begin to chuckle as I hang the chain around my neck. These will deflect unwanted souls and save me from the sun's harmful rays. We had a few hours to kill before our first class so I decided to browse the street shops to find my way to Sandra. When I came back from lunch for school, our class is filling up and I sit at my desk. Its old school animation desk has a hole cut out in the middle of the desk for the light to illuminate the art work through Plexiglas. You could also spin your art work 360 degrees for full control of your pencil strokes. We are lead to a room where we would be sketching people. We take our seats and I sit next to the only girl in class. The instructors go around the room asking people why they chose to be here they finally came to me. Little shy and embarrassed I said that "this was the best thing I could do." The instructor said "ah good answer." After our little intro to our class mates it was time to head home from our first day. Tomorrow we would start our classes and it was going to be intense. We had 6 classes and the toughest one was a 3 year architectural course all free hands crammed into 6 weeks. Few weeks had passed in school and under intense pressure for the load of work we had to do I was slipping faster and faster out of my own reality. The character I was creating for my story that I was trying to make into a short film was of an owl but really he was an angel. Earlier as we had drama classes I was asked to live my character and with my friend Harley standing next to me I pushed him and said "it's all about balance!" With very strange looks on the class's faces the instructor was telling me "that's it?" "I think you need to work on that a bit more." I of course later explained to her it was about an angel and I was trying to bring him to life. She shivered and said brilliance is such a fine line. "Please take your time with this idea Ben" "take baby steppes." nearly overwhelmed with emotion I said thank you, I will. It was now mid-November and our courses finals were coming up before Christmas break. After the break we would be starting 6 new classes, and compiling what we learned so far into them. Today was the final for our drama class and I needed a skit for the final, this skit would be taped. Harley was my skit partner and as he approached the theatre where I was casually having a smoke he says to me "Are you ready dude!" I said calmly "yes." He said "you're sure now you're not going to mess this up this is our final!" I said I have it all under control. But to be honest the more the pressure came with loads of work from the school the more I did my own thing. I was extremely failing every course I had and at twelve grand for the year's tuition it wasn't really the best thing to do. Everyone started to gather for the class. After a lot of lengthy boring skits it was my turn to shine. My character was of course dubbed "Fowl the Owl" and I was an old time owl trying to teach a baby owl how to fly. I of course performed best under pressure and I had nothing prepared so it was basically going to be improving. I got ready to get into character and acted like I was a drunken flying owl. Crashing into people, into the walls and falling over chairs and the desk flapping my arms like I was flying. I went up on a chair and let out a barfing sound with face up in the air and falling over. Of course Harley was supposed to copy everything I did because he was the baby owl. But all he did was fall over. Everyone in the room was applauding and gave me a standing ovation. After that people were saying I should have gotten an academy awarded, I was now dubbed "the Oscar winner." I of course was just trying to get by with my work I was seriously over matched with my art work some people were doing things I could never do, and I was practically down to stick men with my work. All I could do was try and draw out the angel I called "The man in the chair" I was already having lengthy conversations with him, I was always asking for his name. I knew if I could find out his name I could leave him. Vanquish the voice from my ears. He after all was my darkest angel someone who was with me since birth. Something I had to exhume like a cancer in the body. I began to wander the streets every day seeing new things preying when I would see her, the one I longed for. Every day now my mind slipped into a dream state. Not knowing who I was not knowing if I was alive or dead. I went home on the sky train one night. Now so exhausted I wasn't eating much my diet mostly was coffee a lot of coke and the odd sandwich. I wasn't sleeping either, my hours so long and the work load so drastic I didn't know if I was coming or going. I walked to school this morning, I knew what was leading up to my ascension to heaven, and it was going to happen today. I left the station; the sun was dancing between some rain clouds and the buildings above. I could see snow half way down the mountains and I thought to myself the sun is melting the souls of people. We are all going to heaven! When I get to the school I walk up the stairs and see that there is no one there. Angered I leave, confused as to where they went. I storm out of the school and head back to the station. I get to the entrance; I light a smoke and stare at the sun. It's your entire fault I say. I am coming for you! I will know your name! I begin to walk down the streets my body on fire. I take off my coat and my pack that ended up getting shredded was at home. In a rage I start to cut down everything I seen with my eyes, nothing exists anymore! You will no longer burden me! I look up to the tower that was converted into a restaurant and as it spins I had an image in my mind. I had Images of a dark angel above looking down on me over the heavens. condemning me to a life of immortal sins. With flashes of light and my ears hearing high ring tones I hear a voice shout "Bazalzabub." That's it I shouted! That's your name! Laughing uncontrollably I run faster across streets up stares to buildings. I began knocking on all the doors. The faster I walk the more I know I can kill him. I run in the underground mall storming up the escalators and jumping as hard as I can on every floors steel grate. You will never find me Demon! I get up to the top floor of the store and then run as fast as I can down the escalators. In my mind I have opened another dimension. Proud, I walk to a café and take some water. When I sit down in the chair that was free I began to watch the people come in and out. Soon other people were sitting around me. Laughing, cheering, and all smoking, I began to think what I have done is great and everyone can now follow. I close my eyes and see a sword. I hand it to a child in my mind and she dies! Screaming Sandra says "you have killed us all!!" I jump in my chair panicked I run out to the street and its completely dark out. I look up to see the moon and in my mind I see Sandra screaming as she rolls off! I have become unbalanced I thought. Then in an instant I feel a looming presence around the earth and moon. "You have doomed this plain of existence" a voice boomed. I see a halo of light like an elastic band jump from the moon. I begin to walk panicked I can't close the dimension I opened up! I take my ID and buss pass that was around my neck and throw it over a fence, "the sun will never find me" I said. I walked the city streets watching my shadow split in the light of the street lamps. Thinking to me, my soul is splitting. I walk and begin to think Sandra is waiting for me above but I am doomed to dwell on this earth a curse. Walking the streets of the city there isn't a soul to be seen. Everyone is gone, the streets are vacant. No cars on the road. I come to a crosswalk waiting for the light to change so I can walk. I look down the street I see a car lights so I wait. It's a limo, it's her I thought. Stopping for a second the limo speeds off. I am an outcast now I am doomed to walk alone. Thinking to myself I should walk down to the water and cast myself in it. I walk towards the water I begin to think. I can't do this I will not perish. I turn around and walk the way I came. I follow the streets and find a covered entrance I sit there a minute pondering my situation. I begin to cry. I'm doomed I thought I'm a curse of this earth, and in my mind I die inside over and over again. I decide the entrance isn't a good place for me he may come down and strike me from the tower. I begin to walk the streets and as I turn a corner I see the streets are filled with people. The sun is coming up on the horizon and like a wave of motion people's heads bobbing in the shadows. I walk when the sun comes up I feel I have grown wings and a halo. But these are not the same as most people think of them. The wings are like a ball and chain and the halo are my shackles. I begin to walk stomping my feet with every step voices running through my mind like a crowded auditorium. I walk, on the other side of the street I see an old city church made of stone. I walk stomping my feet harder and louder. Then as if someone hit me with a baseball bat on the forehead there was nothing but silence in my mind and in my ears. I walk in daze not knowing where I should be and not knowing who I am. I was Lost among the streets of the city. I approach a busy intersection one of my classmate's runs up to me. "Hey there you are!" he said. Oh h-hello. "Where are you going?" he asks. I say oh nowhere. "Can I come with you?" I ask him. He says sure and I start to follow. But for some reason I panic and start to cry. I better not follow you anymore. He says ok but where are you going. I say somewhere but I am not sure where I'll see you later. Like that I am alone again. I begin to laugh uncontrollably out loud; you will not find me I think. I start to walk faster I walk in front of the school and to the corner I start to throw pennies and dimes at the pubs door across the street. Here's your money you sinner buy yourself a drink! Then I hear my name "Ben!" panicked I run down the street. The calling got louder and shriller and the faster I ran. Sprinting around the corner, I stop hearing the voices and slow my pace. I walk and come across a tall business building and in its lobby is a giant pendulum. Watching it I think to myself I am on a two dimensional plain of existence being shredded by its movements. Then my mind wanders what if I am the man in the chair like a trophy as small as an acorn. In my mind everything around me begins to vacuum to my desk, all existence. I am stuck in the chair taking it all into my soul. Everything sucks into me; my forehead slowly begins to touch the statue on the desk. I am locked in space and time forever in a tomb of ice granite. Frozen for all eternity, Night begins to fall and I think I must go home. Finding my way to the station I get on the sky train, closing my eyes. When I open them again I am sitting somewhere different and I am the only one on the train. Some of the florescent lights flicker as the train fly's down its tracks. I wander off the train and find I am in an industrial part of town. I can see the city lights in the distance like stars in heaven I look at all the towers peaks. Thinking to myself we must travel up the ladder rungs to get to heaven. Sandra and I begin to go up we have children with us and old past family members. When we get through the opening to heaven we see it's just another ladder. What goes up must come down I thought to me. We descended the ladder. I walk my legs in pain and every step feels like a knife is slicing my feet. The more pain I feel the more I walk. I come to a warehouse. Trying to open its door, Of course it's locked and all I see is people hard at work. I jump down the stairs and walk into what looks like a field with a backhoe digging a hole. I walk around the hole and think to myself they are going to bury me like a rabid dog. I walk further and find a creek next to some train tracks. I sit on the edge of the creek and close my eyes. Then in my mind I see the universe explode into white glue. Nothing in my mind but a pasty white glow and in the middle of the explosion there is a single atom made of lead. "Target Acquired" I hear in my ears and with flash of light I sit up thinking they're going to start bombing me with satellites! I start to walk and wander back to the train station. Dark out I pay for my ticket with change in my pocket. I get on and there is no one on and I sit in the back seat. Looking, an image is forming in the back seat. It's a girl, staring at me. I blink and she's gone. I get off the train and stand where the bus should stop. Trying to figure out the time I look at my watch and think. This watch isn't for me! I take it off my wrist and smash it on the ground and toss it in the trash. I find a telephone booth and think maybe my uncle can pick me up it sure is a long ways. Not remembering the phone number I cry and start to walk. I walk up to a pizza parlor next to the bus stop and see the door is being held open by a white chair. This is where god sits I thought and I walked into a mall parking lot seeing my shadow split from the florescent lights. I see my soul split in two and as I walk my other soul crosses the road and walks down the street. Terrified I walk back to the bus stop. I stand to think maybe I should go back on the train. I walk up the escalators and when I reach the top I hear an ear piercing buzzer. Frightened that cops might come and kill me I run back down and stand at the bus stop. I start to cry and I feel the presence of god is behind me. With whooshing sounds from behind me I feel my sins being washed away. A voice says to me "Redemption is the easiest things a person can do." tears fill my eyes and I see in the distance a burger restaurant is open. Thinking to myself I could use a burger, I head for the restaurant. When I get inside there's a bit of a line up and someone drops some change most of it rolling to my feet. I scowl and kick it away. The guy who dropped it says to me "thanks buddy" I say no problem. I ordered two dumb, dumb burgers and sat at an empty table.

Biting into the burgers they tasted fowl like poison and death. I spit it out and threw them in the trash. I leave the restaurant. With an awful taste in my mouth, and I hear a loud horn. Jumping I run behind some bushes and hide. Cars were racing down the street with squealing tires. I think to myself they won't find me here. I decide to get out from the bushes and run down the street. I come to a corner and think ah this house looks interesting I walk up to the entrance door and find it's locked. Then with a squawk a cat jumps the fence and startled I run down the street. Light rain begins to fall and I find myself walking around an elementary school. Each of the overhang lights was bright. I keep walking, she is close I can feel it! I walk down the streets I find myself in a dense rural area. Trying to open the car doors of vehicles as I walk down the street I come across a cab and its doors were unlocked. I sit in the driver's seat, no idea how to hot wire it so I can drive home. I think hmm if I sit in the back maybe I can get him to drive me home. All I find is a pack of gum and I get out of the cab. The strong mint of the gum starts to sting and I spit it out, now with another horrible taste in my mouth I walk along the side of the road to a wooded area. I walk along the road and see a car approaching panicking I hide in the trees they will never find me! The car passes by its lights more luminous than ever. I get out from behind the trees and continue walking. I finally make my way to huge condo complexes and walking along the street I look up. She is up there I thought. Walking I seen a sports car with a red blinking light in it. That isn't for me I thought, it belongs to him! I could never own something so nice. Ending up at a corner gas station like the one I use to work at I went in and bought a coffee and a couple packs of smokes. Trying to drink my coffee inside the busy gas station the attendant soon show's me outside. I wander over to the bus stop on the street and start to smoke. Soon as I light the cigarettes I flicked them on the road there taste so horrible I couldn't stand them. Then like an angel I see the 401 bus. The door opens and I put a pocket full of change in the meter. I take a seat at the back of the bus and close my eyes. When I awake the sun is coming up threw the foggy windows, the bus is filled with morning commuters. I had no idea where in the bus route I was. I scraped the dew from the window of the bus and looked out seeing that we were just approaching to where I parked my car. I stepped off the bus and slipped on the ice nearly breaking my neck. Half frozen mud puddle splashing on my shoes. I arrived to my care and I see it's covered in notes with big felt marker on it frozen from the rain of the night before. The notes all pleading for me to call home, thinking to myself they just want to kill me. I peeled off all the paper and drove off to home. When I got home I saw that the sun was just creeping over the mountains in the distance with clouds like fog of early morning rising to the sky. I went inside to find that no one was home. I crawled into bed and closed my eyes. Opening my eyes I seen the cat face to face with me jumping out of bed the cat tore out of my room. I got dressed and went into the kitchen. Thinking to me my uncle and aunt must have perished in the sun's heat; I light a smoke and used a bowl as an ashtray. Butting the smoke after lighting it and wetting it in the sink and washing the bowl out me got my shoes on and headed for my car. The sun still in the same place when I fell asleep, I stared at it thinking you will never find me! I had a vision of me inside the sun being burned to cinders. I got in my car and drove off. I drove and began to think of my family I seen them all together smiling at me after I have died. Everyone is happy and getting along, I see the one I love standing with them comforting them and my dad who I never knew was there no longer the drunk I made him out to be. I drove and stared at the sun and looking around I seen that the snow still didn't come all the way down the mountains. Over the bridge I went looking at the horizon and thinking the earth is melting in the heat. Staring across the water I wept. I come up to a line up, lights are flashing alongside the road and I drive up to a booth. That will be $4.50 sir. I am sorry I told the lady I don't have it. She scowls at and says "then you will have to turn around sir!" security at the toll pointing me to the opposite direction I was heading too. I turned my car around and off I went again. I began to think what my real dad looked like. Thinking he might just be in the next car ahead of me. Speeding up I pull up to a van and look at the driver. No one I know and I slow down. I drive further to see in my mind the demon that was in my ears. He had my body and face but long greasy curly hair. He had needles for teeth and nails. He Had Cat Eyes smoke coming out of his mouth. Shaking my head disturbed by the image I say to myself in a weepy voice... no..... Thinking of Sandra, her gaze cold now and frightening. Voices were screaming in my ears with the end of my life. I weep and drive. I drive and I have more visions I am on a barren icy road sky is white as well as the ground. Snow fills the pine trees of the empty freeway. In the distance I see a bear approaching. The bear wanting to devour my soul and I see my brother. Anyone who has ever punched a punching bag would survive this. Determined to drive to my real home where my mother Alice lived and my brother Steve and my step father Jerry. I kept on driving. Slushy snow began to hit my windows as semi-trucks sped past me. My windshield filled with mud as I ran out of washer fluid a few minutes ago began to slow my driving skills. I kept driving an orange light appeared on the dash, glowing bright it said E. I was absolutely blazing on the sun now, I thought. It was getting very dark out and in the distance I could see lights. I was approaching the summit toll booth. I came up to the toll and asked the lady if she could break a big bill. She asked me how big of a bill was it; I replied it's a twenty. Rolling her eyes she took the bill and handed me a ten back. I then backed up my car and parked on the side of the toll. Never going through it, I then thought if I got out of my car and went over the snowy bank that bear would find me. I then began to think my mind was a solid led weight. I picked up a penny and balanced it on my tongue they won't be able to blow my mind away now. I sat for a while in my mind I knew I couldn't go any further, so I hopped out of the car and seen there was another car parked beside me. I asked them where they were going they said to "Winfield." I said "Kamloops" can I hitch I ride. The replied we don't have money for the toll. I do and handed them the ten. I only remember seeing a man and he was cleaning out the back seat of his car. The car was filled with trash after he cleaned it out I sat in the front and we proceeded to go through the toll. I looked on the dash written in white out the inscription read. "The lord is my rock" it was in very poor writing. I thought staring at the moon. It sure is, and we rolled into the night. My mother Alice answers the phone in a panic, "Did you find him Robert?" "No we didn't apparently we just missed him, he did come home here but he's gone now." "Ok Jerry and I are on our way to help you look for him, Steve is looking with his friends around town in case he comes here." Gene Ben's grandmother is left at home to answer the phone in case anyone calls. Jerry my step farther and Alice get in the truck and in snow covered night head to the lower mainland. My parents reaching the toll and begin to pay, and out of the corner of Alice's eye she thinks she sees my car. "Is that his car Jerry?" they take a closer inspection of the vehicle. "It is" my mom gasps looking at the snowy embankment hoping I didn't walk over it. They quickly phone Leland and tell them where my car is. Arriving at the toll my uncle and Steve my uncle's good friend go up to the lady in the booth asking if she remembers me. The lady says "oh yeah he asked if I could break a big bill he gave me a twenty." you didn't find that odd my uncle asked, the lady shrugs. She then told my uncle there's cameras here but you can't view them the manager isn't here. Nearly ripping the door from the hinges my uncles says "I want those tapes!" the lady calming my uncle down says "I am sorry sir but you need to wait, I'll call the manager." My mother trying to think where the hell I could have gone says to my uncle "we will head to Kelowna he might have gone there." My uncle said "ok, I'll see what the tapes have on them." My mother and step father head back the way they came to go across the summit connector and head to Kelowna.... After I finish eating the officers open the door. Images of them stringing me up, hanging me by the neck came floating in and out of my mind. Then as the lead me out of the station my family came rolling up to the doors. And we all started to cry. I had no idea why. My parents put me in the back cab of the truck and start to head home. The Light is now coming over the mountain tops. All I heard loud and then faint and then loud again was sirens. I hung my head low, images of me being buried in a shallow grave popping in and out of my mind, with everyone smiling and clapping. I had to dig the hole myself though. They at least gave me a pillow. Then they shot me in the head. Other images came to my mind, I was little boy blue on the moon drinking milk and I hung there by my waist withered and dry with my soul weeping out of me. I was hung out and left to die. Then the truck started to slow down. Thinking this was it for me they pulled into a restaurant that was serving breakfast. "Would you like something to eat Ben?" my mother asked me. Unsure of what I should say I muttered softly "ok." They ordered and as the waitress brought the coffee I seen a skim of light pass from the ceiling to the cup and as I glanced back to the ceiling and it was gone.

Terrified I looked at my family and began to cry. Looking only at my hands with my head down I seen my fingertips were black with grime. I looked at the people all eating and making rather annoying noises in the restaurant. With my perspective everyone was leaning right then left feeling like the place was spinning I said we need to go. Just as the waitress puts down the food, I had no apatite what so ever. Not understanding why we had to leave my parents paid for the food and this time I sat in the front of the truck. We started down the freeway and I see a Cadillac speed by. It was white with tinted windows. Images of god and Sandra sitting in there laughing at me they were saying "your boat sank ha-ha." I slipped in and out of consciousness. We came down the freeway and into the valley where Kamloops was. They drove into town but not to home. I questioned them where we were going too. But neither of them would tell me. We passed the restaurant that Richard and I frequently visited after working a shift at the night club. In my mind I heard a voice say "sorry Buddy!" we headed down a few more intersections and we made our way to the emergency hospital. I was terrified of what kind of experiments they were going to do to me. I said I can't go! But I wasn't given a choice. Through the doors of the hospital we went and they sat me on a bed in the ER.I sat down on the bed of the ER my mother began to take off my shoes, all I could do was stare blankly into space murmuring stuff that didn't make any sense. They took of my ratty shoes and my dirty socks now black but once were white. My feet were bleeding from the toe nails and on both feet there was a single blister bigger than a five dollar bill. I sat there blankly rocking back and forth. My mom left me for a bit and came back with some tea. "Drink this" she says "There's no poison in it" she tried to assure me. Thinking quite the opposite I took a sip then put it on the tray next to the bed. Saying to her "well tastes like there's poison in it!" "they wouldn't let me put any sugar in it" she tried to plead, "Bah" I said "poison!" shaking her head she left it at that. I noticed an old man walking up to the counter I started to laugh at how slow he was shuffling to the counter. Tears nearly rolling from my cheek's I then noticed a piece of tape on the floor. Thinking to me the demon is coming to destroy me. I began to panic, my mother trying to calm me down, saying your brother is coming to see you Ben after he's done boxing" Terrified thinking this is it I am going die Now!" A doctor led me to a room with a chair that had a giant UFO on it. Why am I here I asked. "Oh" a nurse said "we are going to scan your brain" I was very interested in this and thought, neat this should be fun, I bet they find out I am psychic. Laughing at the potential of my brain being scanned I was excited I wanted the results immediately. "How long will the results take?" I asked. "Not for a few weeks" a nurse replies. Dang it! I thought to myself. I found out later when I was recovering, that's standard procedure to scan the brain for any tumors as that is the cause of most psychotic episodes. Luckily for me the results came back as a Negative for any tumors. A nurse came into the room and said ok we are ready to transfer him now. There was a security guard standing with me and they were taking me to a place called One South. At some points during them leading me to one south I panicked and wanted to flee but my mother kept taking my arm and insisting I was to go with them they wouldn't hurt me. They lead me to the back of one south to where they kept the very seriously ill patients. My mother went into the room where I would be staying and began to talk to the doctor. She was giving him parental rights over me due to the fact I was mentally ill. A security guard no older then I sat in a chair by the door. A nurse behind the counter said ok I need you to change into these cloths and please hand over any tobacco you have. I emptied my pockets then changed in the bathroom they had. I came out of the bathroom and handed the nurse my clothes. I say to my step dad "Boy they sure are serious around here aren't they?" he burst out laughing. I paced between the small hospital rooms and looked inside mine seeing the windows were caged and I could hardly see out of them , my mom later telling me you can see in the room from the outside. I sat down in a chair rocking back and forth. The thoughts were racing past my brain. Then down the hall came the dinner tray. I don't know what they put in the food but it was god damn delicious. I ate as much as I could. I wandered into my room and my mom was leaving for a few hours to go home for dinner telling me they would be back and would see me later. When they left I went in my room and closed the door. I put my back against the wall and felt the room spinning out of control. I was looking at my bed and could see the sheets melt into one another back and forth. I began getting nauseated and Closter phobic from the room. I went out of my room sitting in my chair rocking back and forth. Nurse soon brought me some medications. This was an experimental time for the doctors to see which family of medications would keep me balanced. The first drug they gave me was called Haldol. What it did to me was turn me into a zombie. I could only walk as slow as a snail shuffling my feet. My motor skills were greatly hindered and after a few days of barely moving anywhere the doctor decided it wasn't working. The next drug they tried was an experimental drug and when they switched me they were giving me a day pass to go home. When I arrived home all I did was sit in a chair and cry. My grandma started to massage my head asking me of my head hurt. All I could do was nod. I had visions of the big fish in the sea was after me the one they called god. I walked into the bathroom and then was struck down and heard a voice say. "You are now bound by silence!" I wept my tongue couldn't utter a word of speech. My mom and grandmother then decided to take my blood pressure. They thought the freaking machine was broken my blood pressure kept on reading 210 over 52. Worried my mom phoned my family doctor. My doctor clearly stated if you bring Ben here we will phone the police. Not knowing what to do my mom drove me back to one south and talked to the psychiatrist that was handling my medication. They quickly gave me IV and monitored my blood pressure every hour. They quickly switch the drug I was on and tried another experimental drug called Risperdal. Still in a daze from the last drug I woke up in the back of one south and walked out my room. There was an older lady in the room to the left of me. Her door was open and for some reason I walked to the entrance of the door. To me her head looked like a tumor and thinking her brain was the brain of god. Not wanting to but feeling my arms were forced I brought my hands up and palmed my hands in a praying fashion. She says to me "I know why you're here!" muttering I said "you do?" "Yes" she says "your here about my house." Confused I sat in my chair and pondered her answer. Rocking back and forth in my chair I have a vision of Sandra she's standing in heaven with all heavens souls and god. They all start to laugh and smile and condemn me to be the jinx statue in heaven. They place a jester crown on my head and I am deemed the reason everyone will go to heaven and I am left in the cold never to know what it is like to love. Rocking back and forth I begin to weep. I look down the hall and see a nurse with the med tray on her way. Constant beeping in my ears I see a red dot like a laser go from her shirt to the walls to the ceiling and to the floors then vanish. Terrified I take my medication in silence. The nurse at the counter say's to me "Ben you can go to the lobby today if you like." I say happily "ok, thank you." she then says "you can have some cigarettes too." thanking her I start down the hall and head towards the lobby. When I get to the lobby there's a pool table a lot of chairs, drinks for people like decaffeinated coffee. Several people were in robes and such reading books on the sofas. They have a radio playing and a song comes on. The DJ of the station say's "And here's a new song by Sandra" thinking I was meant to be here my destiny unfolding I sit in a chair and began to rock back and forth. Weeping to the music it rips my soul apart. After the song is over I decide to head outside for a smoke. Careful to hide how many I have due to the fact I didn't want to hand them out like candy to the rest of the people in here. I go outside and sit in the tin shed they have for smokers, it was rather cold out only a few more days till Christmas. I sit in there to see a few people there sitting smoking. I sit there rocking in my chair one of the ladies who is in for mental illness say's "I am butting out Satan" another one of them pipes up "that's a good idea! Butt out Satan!" my eyes wide open taking a drag from my smoke thinking they know what I know. Finishing my smoke I go inside for a coffee. There's only decaf though and I load it up with crème and a lot of sugar. I sit and listen to the music on the radio nurses was coming to me and say's "Hello Ben" I say hello and she then asks me if I would like to come to her class tomorrow. I ask what kind of class? She told me it's a crafting class most new residents have to attend it. Its consider part of the therapy process. I say ok not really too interested in it because I was thinking its where most of the crazy's need to go but not me I am not crazy. After a few more coffee's I decide to head back to my room to lie down. When I get back to the back of one south the nurse at the counter says to me "Good news Ben you're being moved into a better room" great full I say *thank* you. They transfer me to just down the hall way of one south to where the more stable residents are. I notice a lot of people are here because they tried to attempt suicide or have what's called Bi Polar, there are also quite a few people with another illness called Manic Depressive. Not really understanding what all this is I walk back to the lobby and decide I'll sit on a sofa and listen to music. I find an empty sofa chair and sit. On the coffee table next to my chair is a pamphlet, the cover had a bob wire outlining a person's head. The title of the pamphlet had the word in bold type Schizophrenia. I opened it up and began to read what it was, then after careful examination I read the symptoms, there's two types of symptoms what's called positive and negative. Not understanding what that meant but after reading the list of what the symptoms were I noticed I had a lot of them. My mother told me earlier that the doctor was leaning to paranoid schizophrenic for my diagnosis. Of course the doctor later explained that the diagnosis isn't set in stone and that it would take over a year to properly diagnose me. I was becoming more stable on the drug Risperdal, and was allowed to go home for Christmas. After a few weeks of day passes and coming more in tune with reality I was release to go home. It was still a rough time for me though I was still stabilizing. I had nightmares of the events that happened to me every night. I had Nightmares of out of body experiences, aliens abducting me and feeling my body being grasped by hands that pulled me through walls. I also couldn't sleep well I would wake up at 3 am look at my digital clock think it's code and pace in my parent's kitchen. Then hours later be so tired I couldn't keep my eyes open. I couldn't stay on a regular sleeping pattern. One of the conditions to my release was I had to visit the doctor every week so he could monitor me. When I went to the sessions I was explained that there is no cure for schizophrenia. More than likely I would be on a disability pension the rest of my life unable to work or go to school. The doctor then explained to me that my illness was probably triggered from me smoking cannabis. He also explained that most people with schizophrenia don't realize there sick they take their medication and after a week of feeling fine they come off them and the chances for a psychotic relapse is extremely high. He also went on to tell me that for some reason smoking tobacco helps to alleviate the illness even though he didn't condone smoking, the fact is 98% of schizophrenics smoke. One of the biggest side effects to my medication he went to explain is weight gain. Not only the illness itself makes me docile but the medication also add to the docile symptoms, which is misinterpreted as laziness by most people who do not understand the effects of the medication and how the illness effects people. There are some areas of mental health that try to help people cope with the illness especially those who don't have families. But the fact is the funding to mental health and schizophrenic societies is nowhere near what it could be very little funding goes into those areas of the health boards. From that I would start my recovery process. It isn't a quick fix it would take a lifetime of coping. I soon found my friends doing their own things that didn't include me of course, there still my friends they just live their own lives with their own problems. My problems were substantially different then there's however. My family decided that it would be best I live at home with my parents. Living on my own with the pension I had would be next to impossible for me, and I had no skills of how to do daily tasks that most people find second nature. I decided to give up my car I couldn't afford all the things that came with owning a car such as repairs, insurance, gas etc. etc. I soon found myself with a lifetime of free time and not a lot to really do; finding things to keep my mind active was a very hard thing to do. I then decided to save for a new computer and learn to play video games. They were about the only thing I could do to keep my mind active. They were almost like positive therapy for me. But still wanting some sort of companionship, but a life time of video games would be a tough task for anyone. My friends all had girlfriends, cars, jobs. I was left with a computer and a lot of time to dwell and think. For a long time I had a lot of regrets about life. What if I did things differently to change my outcome? Knowing I couldn't change my past, I longed for an idea to change my future. I found I couldn't do my art as much anymore. Having a mental illness like schizophrenia I was forced to retire at the age of 22. But being that young not working or going to school most people just thought I was just riding the system. I couldn't put a band aid around my brain and say look I am sick. People seen me as fine and that there was nothing wrong with me. People also told me I should stop taking my medication, but after being stable for 11 years now I can count how many times I have missed my medication on one hand. Some people tried telling me that I had a spiritual awakening. I was tempted to believe this even to this day. I know now even if I did, the medication don't change who I am inside. I still had subconscious thoughts about what if everything I saw came to be and was true to the end of time. I would have a lot of anxiety over this idea. Over the years I began to think and even start to dream again. After all how do you tell the difference between psychotic thoughts and dreams? The difference is my dreams always gave me a sense of hope. Being in that episode there was no hope. All my senses were amplified to such absurd proportions that I couldn't tell the difference between being alive and being dead. I was left to dwell on my situation.

## Chapter 5

My Obsession with Sandra continues, driving my eighty three Honda accord down the freeway from my home in Rayleigh. I put in the CD that makes me drive faster; my collection of her music is becoming almost full. I have stopped listening to anything other than her music, like a calling from within I try to understand what it is that moves me so. It is coming up to the first year anniversary since my trauma of going missing from my art school with a psychotic episode. I am left with over whelming anxiety of not trusting myself. I had a terrified aching of worry of losing control of who I am again. For the past I was trying to figure out, I was beginning to understand how I would survive on a disability pension being paid monthly of four hundred and thirty five dollars. My parents so far have been pretty much supporting me, however with a car, insurance, gas, not to mention I was a smoker. I also had to give my family some kind of money for food and rent. It was becoming apparent that my life was going to be slowing down quite a bit. I was now left with trying to figure out something that I could do to keep me busy for the rest of my life. With the fact that I couldn't get a job nor go to school, I did not know what I could do. At the age of twenty two saying that I am retired sounded kind of strange because people don't retire at that age. To tell people I was disabled in this day and age without some sort of physical impairment didn't wash over to well with people. For one they think you're just a lazy clown, or you're milking the system because you're trying to be a scum bag riding on society's coat tails. My family had become my biggest support tool, I was there biggest dependent. I was driving to town to go to something the government offered as a peer support program. Feeling extremely nervous of what it was going to be like. I kind of felt like a pig on roller skates not really sure of what it would be like to mix with people I thought would be insane like me. I felt as sane as the average working Joe. The peer support group was being held in one of the churches downtown Kamloops, it was mid fall and the weather was rather dry. The snow was melted and the roads filled with gravel from the last big snowfall. The city always used gravel on the streets when we had a lot of snow. I found parking near the church just across the street and seen I was early. Re-learning to drive again was a challenge. The effects of the medications numbing my senses and the fact I had to adjust my visual aspects from the visuals I had from my psychosis. Understanding that things I would glimpse out of the corner of my eyes weren't always there, it was not an easy task while driving. I also had an overwhelming visual of me getting killed in a car accident and being crushed by twisted metal. Churning in my stomach the paranoia of the visuals made me drive with my judgment skewed. Few people started to gather out front waiting for the doors to open, I haven't really socialized with people I didn't know for a very long time. The fact that I gained massive weight from the medication I was on made me feel extremely out of place. The self-image I had before my traumatizing episode was no more and I was left with a body I did not know. I always had a Feeling of being very uncomfortable with whom I was. When the doors opened to the church people started to go inside. I had a nagging feeling I didn't belong because most of these people were allot older then I was. Most they seemed as if they gave up on grooming too. Little did I know that even with my ideals of being clean cut I would soon in later years fall into the poor grooming line. Some of the people waiting outside started to walk upstairs. I went to the front desk and asked what room the peer support was in. the lady at the desk said, "See those people going up the stairs? Follow them that's where there going".....    Smiling I said thanks to the lady at the desk and began to follow these people to the room it was in. a lady approached me and stopped me, I introduced myself and told the lady my mom had called and I was to come to the group. The lady says "hello Ben I am Mindy welcome to Kamloops peer support." "You can just take a seat here and join the rest of the group were making Dream catchers for a fund raiser." as I sat down I sat next to a man with a big orange beard and afro. This man was actually larger then myself, I was not only astonished but impressed even though I was no small guy. "Hello my name is Dean and you are?" "My name is Ben," out of nowhere Dean says, "Hey everyone Ben here wants to get married" I was stunned to say the least. Even though I knew he wasn't referring to him and I getting married I knew what he really meant. In all honesty I did want to get married to someone very much. My main motivation for coming to the group would be to meet someone that I could get to know. Disappointed at the fact it wasn't in the cards, to find the kind of girl I use to date was never going to happen. Embarrassed I just started to make my dream catcher silently and began to observe the conversations that began to entail of how peoples days were going. The majority of them were not going too well. Even though at first I may have judged these people based on appearance and complete superficial on my part. I began to realize these people are no different than anyone else. It seemed I was not the only one to put them in the lens that I did at first, everyone did. I was still jaded to the fact I thought I was better than this but the truth was these people were literally kicked to the curb in life. Getting through their days was a struggle. They only had each other to depend on; I was later told that the funding for such a group was very little. I left the church, I was happy that it was over. Being the new guy always felt weird with me. When the next week came I went, it did get easier for me to keep going. I hopped in my car outside the church, turned on my CD player that was cranking out Sandra's music. Driving home was such a ritual that I would get to the turn off home and couldn't remember passing any intersections on the way. I started to question this, why I couldn't remember the last Five minutes of my driving. I didn't want to tell anyone because I knew soon as I did it would be the end of my driving. When I drove it was like being put into a trance. The music was flowing through my ears. The engine purring as I shifted the gears. The wind whistled out of my window numbing my senses. When I got home I parked in front of the house. I parked on our street parking spot because I had to keep the driveway clear for parents picking up their children. I got out of my car and began to make my way inside. I could see my mom Alice getting her day-care kids ready for when their parents arrived. I went in the house walking up the stairs to the living room and sat on the sofa. Flicking the T.V. on I could hear the kids ruffling there coats. My mom telling all the little wee chatterboxes to get there shoes on. Now that I look back I think this is when my mom really had no more patients. Honestly I don't blame her I think I spent all she had when I went missing. I flicked through the five hundred channels of nothing to watch. My mom had one little girl left to be picked up and she brought her upstairs. I had to put on cartoons, the annoying singing of toddler T.V. It was better than any of the other channels that were trying to either sell me something or reporting on bad news. my mom started to tell me, "Ben we have to talk soon about staying home a little more, you can't afford to constantly go out all the time." my mother began to tell me how much money I was wasting on gas. I began to realized I felt like I was back in high school and the thought of not having Any social life was like amputating very vital parts of my body. I looked at my mom and said "What about peer support? And going to see my friends?" My mom replies with a bit of frustration, "you can go to peer support but you have to stop going back and forth from town so much, it costs too much in gas." I always felt it funny where ever we moved to we ended up either outside of the main town we lived in or somewhere where catching a bus wasn't possible. We lived fifteen minutes from town and the bus only came out this way three times a day. Being paranoid that I would get stuck in town I never caught it. Kamloops was also very spread out, so catching the bus from Rayleigh would take all day to go anywhere. Trying to stay home and not getting cabin fever or becoming insanely stir crazy was going to be something that would take a very long time to get use too. Being disabled gave me pretty much all the free time I could ever ask for. Trying to find something interesting to do during the free time I had was another task that was almost as over whelming as figuring out who I was. People have lives; they work, spend time with the family, go to bed and do it all over again. For me I didn't really have anyone to relate to what I was going through with. Faced with every minute of the day in my own company was something I didn't want to do. My activities consisted when I was at home of writing, art work, listening to Sandra. It also consisted of studying chess from books I ordered from the new book store that opened just recently above the Aberdeen mall. My artwork, writing and listening to Sandra was something I did mostly in the evenings. During the day I was pretty fogy from my medication. Once the sun set it was like I became clearer with how I was thinking. I would start to really dwell on my psychosis and struggle with understanding why it happened to me. Usually this is when I did my best work for writing and art work while I listened to Sandra. I was able to dig deep in myself and channel my emotions. Little did I know this was a natural process I was learning as a coping tool? Years would pass; I would be able to learn to harness this into a sort of fountain to channel energy for my creative work. No one told me that it would be a coping tool but it was something I learned on my own. I didn't realize what I was doing till years down the road. What was once anguish was turning into an unlimited fountain of creativity? The days were getting short this time of year. Dark by four thirty P.M and I was just finishing dinner. Mom cooked Pork chops and rice, one of my favorite meals. I began to gather my faceplate for my car stereo and Sandra's CD's that I would be listening too. taking my coat my mom tells me "don't be out all night please, I worry," reassuring my mom I won't be late I took my coat and headed out the door. Scrounging up as much change I had, I thought to myself I would have enough for coffee under the stars tonight. If you never been in Kamloops. The freeway travels from Rayleigh and it goes to the top of Aberdeen around the entire city basically in a loop. Kamloops is like the intersection of several different high ways going into the interior of B.C., Kelowna, Merit and Vancouver. Almost like a hub in the province of B.C. it is also the location where two rivers that meet to form one. The North Thompson River and the South Thompson River converge in Kamloops to form one river. The Thompson River flows down towards the Pacific Ocean which is later called The Fraser River. The two rivers converging in Kamloops is of high significance to the local First Nations community so I have been told. I jumped in my car and through in Sandra's cd. Pulling the car out of the driveway and made my way to the freeway. Driving from Rayleigh I began to notice there was a star at this time of night shining in the sky. The star would always be directly in front of me facing south. This star wasn't like most stars at was extremely bright and it didn't move like the other stars. For months I had been racking my brain trying to figure out what it was. I knew it wasn't a star or plane so the only other explanation was it had to be a planet. Which planet was a mystery to me? I was always fascinated with astronomy along with my obsession to study chess. Astronomy was a very close second to what I wanted to learn by self-education. For a while now I have been surfing the internet for some sort of telescope to buy but of course with my tastes I wanted the four thousand dollar scopes. In my situation it probably wasn't going to happen, ever. Like a beacon in the sky the planet seemed to follow me if it wasn't in front of me where ever I went it would be behind me. Like an angel looking down from the heavens guiding me. I entered Kamloops and my need for speed was the norm of my driving. My little Honda accord even though not a sports car I could drive it like one with its low center of gravity. I would go there in the mornings to animation school during my psychosis. In Aberdeen they just finished building a new movie theatre and above a huge book store. Kiddie corner built into the book store was Coffee Shop. Whenever I came to this store I always liked pulling right up in front of it. There was never parking upfront it was always filled with cars. When the book stores opened they had a policy that you could sit on a comfy sofa chair find a book, browse it, and then if you liked the books you would buy them. They also had little tables you could put your favorite coffee on. However store policy would eventually change. Removing the sofa chairs because people would end up spending hours there reading books and not buying them. Whenever I walked into the Coffee Shop at this store a wave of nostalgia would come over me. When I was fourteen I was entered into the KMB modelling competition at the Hotel back in eighty nine in Vancouver. I was living in Taber Alberta at the time and after we got back from the competition we would be moving to Kamloops the same day. When I was at the hotel in Vancouver we had to go into different categories at the competition. It was part of the program of showing what you had to offer the many world agencies for modelling. At the end of the competition you could showcase your portfolio to the agencies. My little brother Steve was also part of the competition. Our modelling agency in Lethbridge spent months preparing us for what would be the most exciting time of our lives. When we arrived in Vancouver we decided to start off right. The chaperones with us decided to rent us a couple of limo's to go to the hotel. I was extremely excited, I never been in a limo before. Arriving at the hotel, I felt like this is how I want to spend the rest of my life. Without a care in the world and feeling like I was someone important. The classiness of it all made me feel like I was a very special person inside. During the competition there was a huge buzz at the hotel. Not only were they hosting the KMB modelling competition. The Bent Steel was also staying there while they were performing there Steel Wheels tour. Being fourteen the prospect of being a famous kid was like living in another world made of dreams. The hotel gave me a sense of Class and Elegance that fit the sombre mood of being someone very special. During the competition the conferences were very boring more geared towards late teens, early adults. I was more nervous worrying about when it would be my turn in the spotlight. One of the things we had to prepare for during the competition was doing a scripted commercial in front of a camera. My commercial was about Nike shoes. I loved Nike, I played a lot of basketball in school and all the kids had to have their Air Jordan's. The only thing that was awkward during the competition was my brother and I were sporting the chip and dale tie dyed clothing. For my little brother was ok. Being fourteen and in the midst of a lot of very cute girls. I felt like a dork. In the midst of it all I realized in my head that I was very much dressed like a kid. The fact that I would be in the spotlight in these cloths in front of a lot of people made me cringe. If I wasn't worried enough of being in the spotlight I had to wear kids cloths on top of it. It was just after lunch and our group was being chaperoned into the commercial conference where everyone had to take their commercials and do a practice run in front of a camera and get critiqued. Dreading the moment of performing, I wanted to hide in a hole. What seemed like ages was making me anxious it seemed my group would be the last to perform there commercials. I didn't even care if I screwed up because it was taking so long. Finally my name was called. I walked up in front of everyone a little woozy from the pressure of being the center of attention. The instructor finally said ok you can do your commercial. I started to recite my commercial and without realizing what I was saying or the fact I was under so much pressure I was done. My chaperones jaws dropped astonished at what I did. The instructor said "ok let's look at that on the T.V." Not realizing what had happened the instructor didn't really have anything to say as she watched my performance and said "ok you can go Ben." Puzzled I went back to my seat and my modelling instructor looks at me saying "My God Ben you killed it! That was the best commercial I have ever seen, talk about cracking under the pressure." The conference speaker says "you can go do your real commercial in the other room Ben." I thought " huh, I guess it was good." feeling just a little relief I belt out my commercial for real this time in front of a camera in a closed room. I sat in my chair next to my brother. We were near the modelling instructors and chaperones. It was getting close to dinner time and even as luxurious as the hotel seemed to me, there restaurant was also Luxurious with their prices. Under our budget we had to eat in the malls food court that was connected to the hotel. The mall was huge taking up several of Vancouver's city blocks underground. I was truly raised by my mother because I always loved shopping. I loved shopping even more when I had no money. If I had it, I spent it. If I didn't have it, I would spend everyone else's. My mom tried to teach me the value of a dollar. I always felt if I had it I should share it with everyone. Unfortunately it lead to me begging my mom for money every time I went into the stores. It never ended well when I had to ask my mom for money. Our group ate there mall cafeteria food and went back to their rooms getting ready for the runway competition which would be held in the malls huge foray. They would wait until the mall closed for the night. With the KMB agenda our group would be in the second night of the competitions runway showcase. It also included our photos that we had to get taken as part of our portfolio. There was probably close to four thousand people in this competition. When it came time for the runway, there was a lot of hooting and shouting. All the girls were cheering the guys at the end of the runway. The build-up of when it would be my turn for this part was terrifying. Being in Navy Cadets learning to march the previous five years was a fear that it would be exposed when I did my runway walking. I had to wait an extra day for my runway walk hopping it wouldn't be the duck walk from navy cadets. The pressure was beginning to be so over whelming I had to put it somewhere my mind could deal with. I ended up discovering that it would only be woken up later in my life. The next morning I had my breakfast. I decided to go to the lobby of the Hotel and see if I could spot these Bent Steel people. I had no idea what they looked like and all I knew was they were old. My brother and I hopped into the elevator and headed down to the lobby. When we arrived in the lobby we had seen that it was filled with cameras with reporters and a slew of people from the media. The only place to sit was a couple of sofa chairs next to the corner of the lobby where the hotel stuffed there fake plants. Feeling frustrated with all the hype of the morning one of my chaperones Kim came to sat next to us. "So have you guys seen Ryan Storm yet?" puzzled I said "no, who's that?" Kim looks at me with astonishment and says "you don't know who Ryan Storm is?" I look at her with no thrill in my eyes, "No I don't know who he is." Kim began to explain to me who he was almost as if she was going to start to drool. After a lengthy explanation I said to Kim, "Ok I am going to find this Mr. Storm!" laughing Kim says if you find him I will love you forever. I said "follow me this is the last place he will be." we push our way through the media frenzy and head up the escalators which led to the foray of the hotel. I proceed to walk around the corner of the escalators towards the elevators and stop. I was about to say "well he's not here." We turned around there was about four security guards opening the elevator. Around the corner we just walked a Very short and skinny man in a suite with a plush milky scarf was walking towards us. He walked so fast he turned and went in the elevator and was gone. everyone in the area was blinking with stunned looked on their faces and Kim freaking out, "That was Ryan Storm!!" pissed off that I never had a chance to even shake his hand I said " That little man was Ryan Storm??" he was no further than five feet away from us! Everyone around the elevators on the sofa chairs were mesmerized and started to laugh at how no one had any time to say anything. It was like everyone froze in their spots. Kim was pretty much shaking me like a mad woman at this point. I thought to myself "Damn it!" later I would laugh at that memory at how fast and how frozen we all were to not even say his name. That was pretty much the highlight of the entire trip. After dinner, I was getting nervous at fear of failing in front of four thousand people. I only had one outfit that wasn't tie dyed and it consisted of dress pants shirt shoes belt and tie. The events of the evening began and I was nearly one of the last to do my runway walk. At center stage my pictures were on the movie screen.

The screen was about three stories high. The music started and I began down the runway. My mom and aunt didn't want miss the runway part that my brother and myself had to do. When they entered the mall to watch all they could see in the distance was the movie screen of pictures. My aunt saying as they walked "Oh look there's Elvis on the screen" I finished my runway performance only to have to do it over again. One of the judges wasn't watching me as I performed. I died a thousand deaths to do it over again embarrassed. At the end I walked back to my chair put my legs up and hid my face. After that they showed my commercial to everyone! People cheering and laughing I thought I was the smallest person on earth. I think I even hid behind a fake plant in the mall next to my chair. My mom and aunt found us and said "did you guys see Elvis on that big screen a minute ago?' I said "Elvis? That wasn't Elvis that was me!" my aunt started laughing. Embarrassed I really began to worry now because I looked like Elvis! To lighten the stress I said" Mom we seen "Ryan Storm" my mom and aunt astonished ask what he looked like. I said "I Wasn't expecting him to be really short" my mom laughed. The evening ended with us visiting my aunt and uncle, talking about the fun we were having. The next day, the competition was ending and today would be the day we take our photo portfolio's showing them to various high end modelling agencies. The line-ups for the interviews were ginormous. It was going to take all day to get to display to a few of the agencies. While sitting in line I met a few people who had gotten contracts to some big agencies. I was in the line for the New York agency. Chatting with the New York agents they would set the theme of responses I would get from the other international agencies. "We would like to see you when you mature a few more years and develop a bit more." at the time it felt like my dreams of being a famous kid was shattered but I didn't take too much of what they said to heart. Disappointment at that age is hard to take. The day ended with the awards ceremony. It was a banquette ceremony in the four season's hotel, there was various categories for awards. During the ceremonies my little brother Steve ended up tying for third runner up for his photos. Before we left for the competition because it was so large we weren't expecting to win anything. So for my brother to win for our little group it was a big deal. My brother walked up to the podium and accepted his award. The final category was about to commence and it was the commercials. Of course in my mind I was always critical of myself and never felt deserving of anything. Like my shopping sprees I always felt that the best things in life were only deserved by other people. " Second runner up in the commercial category, Ben Sinclair!" the table I was at all started hollering, "Ben go up there!!" sheer astonishment overwhelmed me and I began to walk on stage with my table going crazy and everyone in the auditorium cheering. I accept the award; I get a photo taken and walk off stage. I sit down and everyone at my table was laughing hysterically , my uncle in tears laughing at me says " Nice sailor walk Ben!" realizing that all crucial behavior I had of controlling how I walked was totally thrown out the door. The duck walk came out of me and was exposed to the entire banquette. In realization of the situation all I could do was laugh with everyone else. After all when you laugh the world laughs with you. When the world is laughing at you, it is impossible not to laugh with them. My modelling instructor reassuring me "its ok Ben that was the true walk of self-accomplishment." the ceremonies were at the end and everyone in the auditorium is being chaperoned outside the hotel. Filling the Vancouver streets with balloons they gave us exiting the hotel. At the beginning of the competition we had to write down our dreams on a piece of note paper they gave us.

With balloons we had we were told to tie our dreams to the balloons and let them float away. Like all dreams we must let them go to be part of the world we live in. after much concentration hoping what I wrote down would come true I let go of my balloon and watched it float away to the night sky. In allot of way's it seemed my dreams already came true. I now had a sense that anything is possible. Little did I know at fourteen what I thought was dreams was a little speck in the events that I would go through later in life. The lofting smell of coffee brought me back to the sensation of those days. The classiness of the hotel, made me feel like I was someone special. The felt special like I was being at peace with innocence. I began to dream to myself, and make a vow. If I ever become a well-known writer I will have a book opening here. As far from reality that was at the time, it all seemed one day it would come true. This time of year Coffee Shop would offer an eggnog Latte. Now depending who was working that night. You would get either a so-so latte or an exceptional one. Not knocking the coffee but it was always a surprise on how much I liked or did not like the latte. Waiting for my coffee at the severing counter, I felt in side of me a sense of purpose overwhelm me. I was being guided to a greater purpose of who I was. What the purpose was and how it would unfold was the mystery of the journey I had to uncover. Like being called to by heaven my works would be the world's greatest treasures. Farfetched it may seem to people the sense of destiny was unquestionable. The sense of fate was my guide as well as my ability to notice the signs I was to follow. The server shouting "Large Eggnog Latte" walking to the counter I took the coffee and make my way towards the books store magazines. They were next to the main part of the Coffee Shops tables. I would walk past the rows of magazines taking mental notes of which ones were written for the good. Only to take notes of which ones were writing foolishly bad. It made a difference to what the purpose I was trying to find to determine the course of actions I would take. I would see that some were interesting, I needed more information. I began to walk deeper into the book store. So sure I was being guided by a divine purpose of great importance. Book covers of the newest books some with covers of where I wanted to be others with covers of a poor inner mood. After browsing the entire store sometimes laughing other times scowling sometimes even nearly crying. I remember why I came to the store. One of my obsessions was trying to study chess, even though I wasn't at all a good chess player. The game itself fascinated me. In my mind if I have to stay home all the time, I was going to use it studying something that would further a self-education. Making my way to the game section I look for the chess books. I see I already have the copies of the chess books there selling. I went to find a store clerk and I ask her if they will be getting any different chess books in the store. The clerk began to explain to me that they only carry a few. If I wanted to special order some I could use their computer kiosk to order any kind I wanted. Interesting I thought this is new; apparently they had it tied to their internet web site. I thought wow guess I can really stock up now. I made a list of the books I wanted and wrote the prices down on note paper they had there. Doing the math in my head if I didn't buy anything for myself for a month I could afford one book a month. And the size of the selection they had. I knew it was going to take me a really long time to get all the books I wanted. I put the list in my pocket thinking maybe I could get mom to cave on buying me some more books. I did learn how to read chess notation but the hardest thing was working the moves on the board. That was another shopping quest I had in finding a decent chess board with notation on it. It then donned on me I should look at the astronomy section of the store to see if I can find out what planet was following me! I made my way to the astronomy section and began to browse the books. Now the reality check comes in. the actual truth was I didn't really read books. I just liked books and I like looking at the pictures. In fact when I tried to read the sound of the words were so painful in my head, the nuance of reading more than one page drove me so insane it was torture. I couldn't sit still more than five minutes without getting antsy to actually finish a few pages. Most of the books in the store were table breakers. It wasn't that I didn't know how to read, I could read quite fluently. It was the process of reading and sitting still that drove me insane. Yet I was determined that I would study chess and astronomy anyways. After looking over the books I didn't see anything that resembled the planet I was looking at. I mean really how I could tell without a telescope. I looked on at the endless pages of words in the astronomy books. Some of the words on the snow white paper would be bold and highlighted while others would shrink and dull out. The words bold and glowing together made no sense when putting them together. Each book had a hidden message I was determined to figure out. What a perplexing circumstance this is I thought. The actual irony of the entire situation we are in riddles me so. I could feel my face getting closer to the pages. With a jolt the realization of the last few sentences of the book I had in my hands became my awakening. The words echoed in my mind and heart. I put the astronomy book back on the shelf asking myself did what just happen really happen. I began fearing that the demons were speaking in my head. Strained my ears filled with the words in my mind. Questioning the messages I was tormented on. How do I put what happened to the words in my story to make it tangible. After all this is what it's all about isn't it? I had to tell people of the state of others living with schizophrenia? What they deal with every day? Or was it more about bringing heaven to earth following the path I was on to make a source of universal awakening... I became entranced with a feeling. Like I was going to die, the exotic feelings of following heaven were just as intensely met with realizations of my own mortality. With a sense of expiring I began to walk out of the books store. It was close to the end of the week and my friends with their work schedules only had the odd weekend to do things. I use to be able to hang out with them daily. After my hospitalization I became aware that I too once worked all the time and it usually seemed like I spent more time with my friends. But with everyday being retirement now, my friends and I seemed to go our separate ways. Another major factor was I didn't know how to have good times with my friends if there was alcohol or pot involved in order to have fun. With my medication drinking anything made me sick and pot was extremely out of the question. When those things become part of daily life it is nearly impossible to become comfortable when it's in your face. Trying to have fun but not being able to participate was something I didn't know how to do. The sad reality was I needed to do a personal change in order to realize that I could be comfortable in the situation that those things were going to be consumed. It would take me years to find that comfort zone but the presence of pot for me was an absolute trigger. I would never be comfortable again being around the substance. Panic attacks were quite common after being out of One South. The thing about panic attacks is learning to recognize you are in fact having one. But somehow try to figure out a way to cope with them. Sometimes it's best to tell someone that you feel one is occurring until you can cope with them using your own tools. Walking out of the bookstore I unlocked my car, adjusted the seat while turning on the ignition. I pull out of the parking lot to make my way back on the freeway. Looking at the time, it's about eight thirty. Traffic at this time was busy outside Aberdeen mall. Christmas was just a month away and the closer it got to Christmas the busier the town became. Mom was so upset of me being in the hospital this time last year that she told everyone that we wouldn't be celebrating Christmas. She said she needed one year to just rebel and not celebrate Christmas. I guess it was her way of coping with my trauma. To me I was so much in a delusional state it never really sank in of what it did to my family. It pretty much devastated them. With schizophrenia being a lifetime disability, it was going to be a long road for everyone in the family. I pass the Aberdeen mall hugging the corner that lead to the freeway. I began to have the sensation of impending doom. In my mind a Giant Grand Piano was going to fall from the sky and crush my head. A vision of me getting in a head on collision was making me sweat. I began to gasp for air rolling down my window. The only thing I could do was start to breathe deeply and try to somehow calm myself down. One thing I learned to do was "Be" with what I was feeling. This would be one of the biggest tools I would learn in my recovery. I would begin to feel every part of my body and ask myself why I feel this anxiety. Nearly crushing me at the time with me wanting to jump out of the car and get torn up by the pavement. I drove home well under the speed limit. Driving home I would watch every car that passed with caution. I reassured myself I was driving on the right side of the road. Finally making it to Rayleigh, I was turning off the freeway and fear struck me. I began to visualize what if when I cross the tracks I don't see a train but there is really one there? Images started to fly through my mind of being hit by a train. In the carnage that ensued I would be disembowelled and dismembered making a bloody mess for someone to clean up. Nearly making myself sick I sped so fast over the tracks I think the car left the ground. My heart racing I take the corner and drift home to the spot in front of the house. I quietly enter the basement entrance where they day-care was and head upstairs. I felt calmer because I was in a safe environment. I walk upstairs to my room toss my jacket with my car stereo faceplate along with the cd on my bed. I took my black sketchbook and my Walkman with a tape of Sandra's music. I walk to the living room sofa chair. Turning on the lamp I decided to thumb through the pages of my pocket sketchbook. I had a lot of pages of writings I did in the hospital. I can remember I did a lot of writing while I wandered the streets of Vancouver. None if it made sense and it seemed as if it was some sort of message from heaven. My brain was trying to figure it all out. I put an absorbent amount of stress on myself that whatever it was it had to be perfect. In stone cold reality how do you make gibberish perfect? The only one it meant anything to was me alone but I knew the message was meant for everyone. I guess with this understanding I felt like the only one on earth who felt as though there was more to what we are as people. Yet as outlasted from humanity as I felt, one day what I was going through would make sense. What I had to say would change things. The irony of trying to separate my Dreams from my Delusions was part of what I needed to process as a person fighting schizophrenia. What was the difference between the two? Was my dreams so different then my delusions? Was what I considered unattainable in reality possible? The odd of me being successful was impossible to fathom. If I were to be successful in what I envisioned would it truly be the work of heaven? Every possibility flashed through my mind as I continued to write about what I seen. Then the question came to me that I feared. What would happen if I was a success? In my mind it would mean I would be dead. Fear is what usually kept me silent in telling people what I seen. When I describe the things I see with my family it in turn gets dripped into the conversation with my psychiatrist. Who in turn writes it down in his note book? Fearing the authorities to prescribe drugs that make my senses disappear and the ability to process thoughts become dull. The pills would make my ambition to get through the day slowing to the point of being lethargic. Some things are best left unsaid. When society is fear based it can condemn people for "Acting" different then "Normal. "Like paranoid people fearing paranoia. There are two possibilities of what happens after being faced with psychosis. The fact it usually happens in young adulthood, it goes like this. You either become a recluse or you have an unquenchable thirst for companionship. I had the thirst for companionship. The whirlwind of what people experience in this situation eventually seem like acts of desperation. At least it did for me; there was nothing more painful to me then the feeling of not belonging. That feeling was amplified to my feelings that I was not human. In my mind trying to not only cope with delusions but insatiable emotions for companionship. It was unbearable to deal with at times. The only thing that helped to cope at the time once the sun went down. When the vampire in me began to stir was writing or painting. The longing I felt to one day be recognized as a significant writer or artist was enough to fulfil myself. Thinking that I might not be accepted today or belong in society now. "But one day I will be" more accepted then I could possible desire. I took hold of that dream that "One Day I will be" and it in a way gave me the comfort in knowing that I had it in me to accomplish anything. I had the strength to take on anything that was set before me. The feeling of one day I will have all the answers I ever asked for. It was the foundation of my recovery. I put my sketchbook on the coffee table of the living room and sat back in the chair tuning off the lamp while listening to Sandra. I closed my eyes and tried to feel what I was feeling with my emotions. The weight of anxiety was one feeling in my body. The noise in my mind couldn't be quitted but instead I would let it turn to white noise. In my head was where I would get the sensation of hearing but what I was hearing was just static. This started the sensation of time standing still in the darkness. I was just "Being" where I was at that present moment. This was very new to me, so being the first time I tried this it was taking a lot of concentration. Keeping everything the way it should without being swept up with what my mind was making for me. Controlling the things I would see and hear. Bring with the weight of trying of anxiety takes a lot of practice. It's not easy to not let it go where it wants to go. Then trying to keep it where it should be. Being aware of where it sits in your body the feeling of where the weight feels the heaviest. With me concentrating on the sensations I turn my palms face down and start letting it flow towards the ground. First it felt as though my innards were going through my feet. Once I began to do this more often it became easier to understand what was happening. I soon would fell asleep. My nights would be restless the medication was rough at first. Trying to find balance with the medications and the things I was going through was rough. It would take a few med adjustments and adding another which was a mood stabilizer to find balance. My mom's "No Christmas" went off without a hitch but after it was over she made another vow. It was to never miss another Christmas ever again. Over the next few years my social life really came to a grinding halt. Losing touch with most my friends I was now spending time with my cousins and aunt. My panic attacks began to be well controlled I hardly had them anymore. Although learning to deal with them was always two steps forward one step back. My out of control emotions with the delusions were starting to subside to the point I forgot about what they felt like. But I always remembered what they were about and could still see them plain as day. Along with the subsided symptoms I use to have, now it was just about getting through the days as best possible. Trying for a better quality of life, rather than if I was not on medication. My family was the cornerstone to my long walk to recovery. It seemed no matter the situation I always had a place I could call home. The years that followed though were not without its tragedies. First my aunt's husband died of a drug overdose. It devastated my cousins, all of them were just finishing high school or within that age range. The year that followed was quite rough, but it wasn't long after that my aunt died from the influenza. Now my cousins were left with no parents. They had to rely on each other and what seemed like I string of bad luck got worse, well for me at least. I had a friend who I went to peer support with. He was stricken with schizophrenia much harder than I was. If you were to look at me and talk with me you wouldn't be able to tell anything was wrong or that I was disabled. With my friend you could tell something just wasn't right. My friend ended up not taking his medications for a week and was slipping into a deep psychosis. His medications to me were extreme. I was on very low doses of two different medications. My friend had more than nine different medications. After a week he missed his medication. My friend was alone in his apartment and panicking he had taken an entire weeks' worth. He then proceeded to drink a full bottle of sake. I received the call from my friend's dad that my friend had passed away. The call so surreal, bounced off me like a bullet off bullet proof glass. These events would take the questions of my mortality to their peak. Unable to deal with how I felt I was numb. His death was called an accidental suicide. When they had his funeral, I couldn't bring myself to go. My mom, brother and grandma attended. During the funeral there was not enough seating for all the people that attended. My buddy had made a lot of friends that accepted who he was, regardless of any condition he may have had. For me though I decided I wouldn't pursue any more of my writings. I let go of my artwork and packed up all the supplies I had. Taking all the music I had of Sandra and tossing it in the trash. I told myself that I would not follow the same path of my friend. I would not be just another statistic to an illness that consumes people. Giving up my obsessions was a reality of being part of the illness. I now began to stay home and just work on the computer playing online games. I was told a few months down the road that the funding for the peer support group had been cancelled. While I was going to peer support, I managed to get on disability two which was allot better and gave me double the money I was usually getting. Unfortunately I had a habit of ordering things online that kept my visa constantly a couple thousand dollars in dept. it would add to my cost of living with visa payments. I was left with around hundred dollars extra a month to spend on what I wanted. My mom would in the next year close her day-care and we sold our house in Rayleigh. We moved to my uncles in Surrey, my parents spending a few months looking for a place to live. My room at my uncles was in his unfinished basement. I would set up my desk along the wall near my bed, where I would put my computer. With my symptoms now managed by medication. The online gaming was the only thing keeping my brain active on a daily basis. I began to change my focus to the inward journey of discovering who I was. The urge for companionship was now turning into a need of understanding why I was the way I was. I knew deep in my heart that I couldn't love anyone until I finally loved what I was. The hardest part was being with my emotions and how I felt inside taking the step back and observing. Whenever I felt my anxiety it was a weight of hate and rage. The question I would ask myself when I would feel this rage was why? Nothing in my life gave justification to feel this angry. I would have this heavy feeling that had absolutely no justification. I was able to begin to let it go. This gave me a sense of presence within myself. Honing this practice would leave me in a constant state of "being" in the moment. While I began to do this at first I had no frame of reference to what I was doing other than a constant search of asking why. My parents would end up finding a town house in Chilliwack. That summer we moved into our town house complex. Moving from my uncles took several days and settling in new surroundings always would take a lot of time to get use too. The only privacy for me to smoke would only be at our back ground level small patio. We had a very small back yard and the highlight for me was I didn't have to mow the grass. We had a town house tight on both sides of us; luckily the people who moved into them were nice. We bought the town house brand new as it was being built we were excited to be its first owners. From here it was a new beginning, a new time to start fresh but this would not be the end of what would be a recovery. The road is still long, the fight on-going, I would find out what it means to be who I am but the search for myself will be in the next awakening.....

## Chapter 6

I open the patio doors to our town house walking outside, it was a light drizzle from the overcast skies. Lighting my cigarette I hear peppy chirping from above me. On top of a tall tree close to the freeway near our house was a bald eagle and its mate sitting, gazing over the houses. The eagle had built a nest there years prior and was on a route they would fly from the river that was a few kilometres away. The last few weeks I thought I would change my pace by being more active. I was getting ready to go to the Cheam View Club House in Chilliwack. I bought a cell phone last month and was eagerly waiting to add new friends to it. I became recluse while living in Chilliwack and I very much wanted to find people I could relate to instead of sitting on the computer day in and day out. Nervous I finished my smoke and walked inside taking my jacket. Mom was getting ready and I made my way to the garage and got in my mom's car. Driving to the club house didn't take very long even though the club house was on the other side across town. On the way listening to the local radio station one of Sandra's songs came on the radio. Irritated I ask mom to change the channel, or turn off the radio. Rolling up to the club house I can see it was in an old house across from a church. I took a bag that had a bag of French roast coffee in it that I bought as an icebreaker for the people that go to the club house. My mom left as I walked up the stairs to the door of the old house. On the veranda of the house were people sitting in chairs talking I saying hello as I opened the doors. Walking in I could see a kitchen straight ahead an off to the right was there cafeteria. There was different posters and poetry posted on an info board next to the phone in the hallway. Observing the people in the club house I was reminded of the people I went to peer support in Kamloops. Only a few of the people seemed to be close to my age. As I walked around I met up with one of the workers, her name was Janet. She began to introduce me to people and took me on a tour of the club house. I gave her the bag I was carrying with the coffee and she handed it to one of the club house members. When the person looked inside he began to shout profusely thank you to Janet as if she bought it for him. Janet finally explaining I brought it for everyone, he ran and started to brew the coffee. I blushed but was embarrassed at the amount of excitement over the coffee. I met with another worker named Jon, we went into one of the rooms upstairs where they began to tell me the rules of the club house and had forms for me and my doctor to fill out. Telling Jon what I had in mind of what I wanted to accomplish at the club house, that I was looking to network a bit and somehow bring my artwork to the clubhouse to find a way to become recognized. Jon amazed at my enthusiasm asked to look at my work and when the next time I come to the club house if I could bring some. Excited I might be able to get some sort of recognition I agreed to bring some for him to look at. In retrospect it seemed the funding for people with mental illness was a lot rarer here then it was in Kamloops. In the back of my mind thug I was more hopping to find someone I could relate all my stuff too. Someone who old understand who I was and I would be able to open up to the past few years of what happened to me. Feeling awkward I sat for a few hours outside smoking watching the people at the club house, hoping to find a new friend but very shy to the people who were there. Jon coming outside began to tell me about a youth program they had that every Thursday and Tuesdays they would go out and do things with the young adults who were members. Telling me transportation would be provided afterwards but I had to meet at the club house to come I would tell him die have to discuss it over with my mother and then I would get back to him.

I phone my mom telling her ready to come home. Waiting out front smoking I see my mom coming down the road and hope into the car putting on my seat belt. I told my mom about what happened about the coffee she laughed, and told her about young adults. I showed my mom the forms I needed to give to my doctor. We had a new family doctor when we moved down to Chilliwack, he was really nice. That night I was out smoking on our patio and I was watching a satellite crossing the sky. The satellite was bright and I was amazed at how fast it was going. Watching the light cross the sky it all the sudden turned south, I couldn't believe what I was seeing. Then it went behind some clouds, blinking I was astonished then where it disappeared I seen it come back north and fly over top of us. I ran inside scared as hell telling my mom I seen a UFO. My mom knew about the dreams I had before about aliens drilling in my teeth and back and she assured me there was no such thing as aliens and I probably just seen a jet plane. Never the less I cringed at the thought of being abducted. The next day I phoned Jon telling him I would be attending the young adult group this coming Thursday, pleased he let me know when I had to be at the club house and that we would be going to a hockey game. Today I was heading out with my mom to do some shopping in Langley. Our first stop is to pick up my grandma at my uncles house. It was pay day for me so I planned on buying something but what I wasn't sure. I also had to buy my months' worth of cigarettes which coasted about two hundred and sixty dollars; it was defiantly not a cheap habit. Our firs stop would be our doctor's office to drop off the forms. Afterwards we headed to the mall to look around, my grandma wanted to go to the bay to get some new perfume. Walking through the store we approach the perfume counter and like a fist to the face the flowery smells of all the perfumes lofted over the counters. Waiting for my grandma to get her new perfume I begin to wander into the mall. Not far from the bay in the mall was a science and toy store. In the store they had telescopes puzzles and games for educational toys. I browsed the scopes and chess sets they had, the scopes too expensive for what I culled afford to pay. My obsession for collecting chess sets was hard to deny buying one. Mom saying "you're not buying any more chess sets Ben" as I rolled my eyes and put the one I wanted back on the shelf. Leaving the store and walking down the mall hallway I could hear Sandra's music coming over the mall radio. Frustrated I thought I was cursed now I no longer chased her music however her music is now chasing me. Trying to not listen and looking for something that would distract me I continue walking through the mall with my grandma and mom. Walking through the mall there wasn't a lot more I was interested in and after my mom and grandma had gotten there lottery tickets we made our way back to the car and proceeded to our next stop. The next stop on our shopping spree was Costco to pick up my cigarettes. Taking a buggy for my grandma to walk with we walked through the doors showed the Costco employee my mom's card and walked past the T.V.s, Computers, and other electronics. During this time Costco had Apple products and they had displays for the first generation of iPod Nano's. Walking past them I thought this might be interesting but I would have to find some sort of music to listen too, for the past few years all I listened too was the local radio station. Passing the clothing and books I approached the music part of what they offered. As I looked I seen they had one hundred CD collection of various classical music. Showing my mom and telling her about the iPod, mom thought I should get it. putting the CD's and iPod in the buggy grandma asked me "What's an iPod?" it would take me the rest of the day trying to describe what an iPod was and how it worked but my grandma couldn't fathom what it did holding all the music and how small it was. After we bought our groceries there was a runner who had to take my tobacco. I usually bought 4 cartons a month which was extremely expensive. We left Costco and headed for our last stop of the day, to get my hair cut from my cousin Lori and to have lunch with my aunt Susie. I haven't seen my cousin in a very long time so I was happy to visits with her while I got my hair cut. She of course was cutting my hair so I looked cool. Meeting up with my aunt we had lunch at white spot restaurant that was close to my cousin's salon. I was eager to get home and start putting my music on my new iPod. playing with the iPod at lunch my grandma looks at it, saying " this is something I would just throw away if I didn't know what it was." blinking I said " you're not throwing away my iPod!" after lunch we dropped my grandma back at my uncles house and my mom and myself made our way back home. After a few hours of putting the music on my new pod filling it up I spend the rest of the day listening to the great classics. That evening I fell asleep listening to my new music. I begin to dream flying through the forest over log cabins and making my way through the cities I live near. I landed on the street below. The night lights distorting my shadow as I walk. Looking up I see Sandra walking down the street towards me. Walking by our eyes meet and I walk past, continuing down the street. I began to wonder if at all when she looked into my eyes if they did tell her everything. That out of what they had to say, if she knew the pain I was in. I awake my gut wrenching at my dreams images and the daunting cold reality setting into my mind. She does not know me; she is just a person living her life. I begin to be disgusted and sickened by my obsessions. I realize that whatever my thoughts are, an illness and a sickened fantasy I have created. I felt as though I awoke with a hangover. My eyes heavy I make my way downstairs brewing coffee and heading out the door to the patio for a smoke. Over the fence in the field that was once mostly bushes has been cleared to make way for the condo complex that a construction company was going to build. Un-easy that my privacy what little I had would soon disappear. Like a zombie I make it through the day and before dinner I began to get ready to go to the club house for young adults. getting dropped off at the club house I see there's a few people at the door to the club house and I introduce myself. Jon was gathering a few things and we were all about to jump into the club houses passenger van to get the other young adults in Abbotsford and Mission. Once we picked everyone up we had to head back to Chilliwack to the coliseum for the hockey game. Sitting in our seats we had taken up two rows near the cement stares in the building where the hockey game would start. We wear at the far side of the arena close to where the opposite teams goalie was. Once the players were in position and the game began, out of nowhere the quietest kid in the group began to shout obscenities and heckle the away team's goalie. Jon and I were in shock at the words and how loud this kid was, it was extremely funny but somewhat embarrassing. The heckling of the goalie lasted the entire time the away team was at that side of the arena. Laughing to myself at the end of the night I was happy to head home. Over the next few months I would go to the club house once a week and socialize a bit but as I did I began to realize that I wasn't any further ahead in my artwork or making friends and I began to decide that I no longer wanted going to the club house. While I was there I was elected to start an art club and was put in charge in teaching people that wanted to on how to do art work. I did in fact wanted to teach but I hadn't considered myself a great artist and what people wanted to do was beyond what I was capable of. The daunting stress of perfection was so overwhelming I couldn't continue to teach people and son after that I stopped going to the club house. The people I met no longer kept in contact and I was left again sitting in front of my computer a recluse in the town house where we lived in Chilliwack. The condos they were building were finally finished. There was a group of people in one condo that would through parties every Friday night and they would constantly have people sitting on their balcony that looked down at our back yard. Disgusted with the fact of what I use to do and missing all the party's I went too. I decided that I would no longer feel like my privacy was invaded and told my mom that I was quitting smoking. My mother phoned my brother that evening and discussing my want to quit smoking my brother suggests staying with him to help, he was never a smoker and it might be easier if I was away from my surroundings for a while. I agreed and over the next few days I began to pack some things. I was planned to stay for a couple weeks and over the weekend my mom would be taking me up to Kamloops. My mom making very clear that I needed to stay on track with my medication worried she made my rather promise I wouldn't miss any of them. I tried to quite before once after high school and the longest I lasted was six months before caving and starting again due to my mind playing tricks on me. I was hoping this time I would be able to quite for good. The trip to my bothers was uneventful, and when I got there I unloaded my baggage into his spare bedroom. My brother wanted to show me how to cook dinner the way he cooked it mostly a vegetarian dinners. Getting use to veggie dinners wasn't hard but I was irritable from not having a cigarette for the entire trip up. The only thing that would help me quite and it has always been the only thing was Nicorette gum. Patches never worked the Zeeman pills were not an option even though I tried them before they made me get very ill. My brother explained I would have to find something to do while he went to work during the week but my brother lived right downtown Kamloops and I told him all I wanted to do was walk all over town. My brother thought that was one of the best things I could do. Being the new age hippie that he was I knew I would be in good hands. Talking with my brother and explaining to him about what everything I have thought up to this point with my exceptional experiences. My brother began to tell me about enlightenment and how the universe worked. I told him all I wanted was to figure out what I went through meant and why I went through what I did. I told him I longed for something that brought purpose to what I did and that I needed something tangible to hold onto. The next piece of advice my brother told me was the beginning of self-realization for me. He told me what I needed was a mantra a saying that I could say over and over again. By saying this mantra it would allow the universe to bring to me what I was looking for. The tricky part was I had to come up with my own mantra it had to be something personal and I had to be great full for whatever it was I was asking for. Like a riddle to me I started to wonder what it was I was grew troll for. What was it that I wanted more than anything? I asked myself this over and over again for a very long time before I would find the answer. The next few days had past and I was getting my bearings walking around Kamloops. The one great thing about my brother's place was even if I didn't sleep well I could go for a walk anytime day or night. And I took advantage of this Kamloops was a very safe place that I was comfortable with, I knew the surroundings very well. While I was at my brothers I met up with some old friends, I spent a few days with them visiting and even though they were smokers I never caved to the urge of smoking. Spending the time I had at my brothers soul searching I came to realize there were two key things I wanted for myself. One was forgiveness towards me and who I thought I was inside of me and all that it entailed. The second thing I wanted more than anything understood, and that's when I discovered what my mantra would be. Walking in the middle of night across Kamloops I threw my arms up to the night sky with stars twinkling and I said to myself, "I am grateful for Understanding." The more I said it the more the world began to open up and I began to realize the things in my life that didn't make any sense at all. The pain that was so overwhelming in my heart I began to step back and realize the feeling in the presence of forgiveness I began to feel the pain lift. The pain was lifting and for once in my life I began to smile from the inside of myself. The next few weeks at my brother I began to understand that in fact who I was buried with pain and fear of things that were made up in my mind of personal anguish. The knives people said my entire life began to heal and the hole in my heart no longer would bleed for things made up of what I thought were situations of ridicule. The door for enlightenment and inner peace was now opened and I began to see things with a new look on life. But it still wasn't without taking two steps forward and one step backwards, like all things it was like riding a bike one moment you grasp freedom and after that your left wondering how you did it. leaving my brothers with my new insight I would practice this over and over again in my mind deciphering everything that I was and what things meant to me. One of the most significant things I discovered was that to understand god and love one must understand what it is to suffer or be in suffering. To understand suffering is to understand what compassion is. Without compassion people would be left to extinction. This realization turned everything I was going through into something beautiful. And then I realized what my mantra was. "I Am Grateful to Understand." and this realization unto myself brought me inner peace. But like anything this would take time to be at this place. 6 months after being at my brothers

I began smoking again due to inner frustrations. We would end up selling our town house, to move to Chilliwack Mountain. This would be our final move to date. After settling there I decided to pick up my writing once more twelve years have passed since my hospitalization. I never had a relapse into psychosis. I decide to take up my art work as well and questioning why I was so obsessed with Sandra I begin collecting her music again. I send writings to different places all being rejected. One day Jon from the club house calls me up and wanted to meet with me. I oblige and we meet at coffee shop. He begins to tell me about cores the club house is offering. It's about training people to be peer support workers. Interested I tell him I'll take the cores. While attending the cores I discover what it truly meant, to be a peer support worker you have to be in recovery of a mental illness. This statement brought such a self-realization to me that I never knew before. And it was this. I Am Recovered From Schizophrenia. awakened I see that what I kept saying to myself over and over, "I am great full for understanding" has finally come full circle. Amazed at the long road it was I see what I was meant to do. It was just a window into a little room. The journey hurt like hell. But like all journeys it will never end. The only difference is that I know what the purpose was. Listening to Sandra I understand what she was for me. She was then and will always be my Muse to tap into the well of creativity that I possess. Her music is a gift, following me like an angel. Now fifteen years later I sit in my family's doctor's office with my zip drive to my book. I wonder will this be the right place it should go. Will this be how I finally tell my story? Filled with doubt I sit and wait. Like an angel on the radio I hear Sandra's music come on. Why now? Why here? No more of a coincidence then it was fate. Will my story be told? Will people understand what it means to suffer with schizophrenia? people seem to think if you have schizophrenia that you are a murderer and killer, or that when they meet someone with schizophrenia they need to be put away somewhere out of society. the truth is this we are human as much as anyone else is, only during psychosis we are extremely sensitive to everything around us so sensitive to emotions and feelings, that it can make us delusional lost on a trance state. Think for a moment of having all your senses on overdrive yet you are not in your body you're in the place where ever it is that the angels or god has taken you. When I went missing from the Vancouver Animation School I remember bumping into one of my class mates. He asked me the question hey what are you up too? Such a simple question that I could not answer, then he asked me where you are going. Again I could not answer him. All I could do was muttering and cry and in a few minutes of him in my presence I ran away as fast as I could. To me I was scared out of my body. It's been a long time since this has occurred, my trip along the path to god or rather the path to what I thought was good that turned to the road to hell, was something I need to share with as many people as possible. It's almost ironic that if I were to have a voice it's for people who suffer with a stigmatic illness whose voices are not heard by people in their lives, but to them they hear the voices of ghosts and souls who never let them call for help. Most of the time when the onset of psychosis sets in it feels natural and uplifting to the point of euphoria. People will chase this feeling until it breaks them within themselves. Once they are broken, they are in fact are being lead to their actions or their thoughts to the voices that they hear in their head. It's this loss of control that people seem to fear. It is unfortunate that people living with schizophrenia are more likely to be a victim of a crime rather than to commit a crime. here is one of the biggest miss conceptions about schizophrenia, most people either from the medical profession or from family will say you will never recover from schizophrenia, in some cases it's true, but most of the people who do not recover either, A. smoke pot or do some form of narcotics, or do not take the medication they are prescribed. When I was admired to the hospital in one south, most of the NEW drugs were breakthroughs, but had terrible side effects. For me even though this was the case, I would do anything to not be in the state of obsessive mind that I was in. I no longer wanted to fight something I could not control, and be tortured by my own thoughts. There are 2 things someone with the trauma of early schizophrenia must do. Understand that it is possible to recover, and have the insight that the medications are infect there to help stop the tormenting thoughts that come with schizophrenia. It takes a lot of self-insight and acceptance that it's a process of understanding what the illness does. It takes people to choose to understand what it is there going through and to not stop the medication once they feel better. If they stop the medication the "feeling better" is temporary. Here is the major niche about the reason for someone with schizophrenia to not take their medications. Schizophrenia affects the part of the brain that deals with religion. The major factor to religion is being pure. So in fact being medicated goes against ever part of our soul for we feel we are not worthy of the blessing we receive, even though it's an illusion. However on the other hand you could say god gave us a brain to think of cures for illnesses, so in fact we would still be loved by god regardless. The one thing that kept me safe, like an angel that was with me through all my illness, was Sandra's music. it's the only thing I can think of that kept me from being killed or never coming out of the darkens I was in. it seems that most people who develop schizophrenia have an above average IQ. I tend to think I just made bad choices growing up that led to my downfall. But even today I still listen to Sandra's music when I paint or write. I tend to think one ay somehow or some way she will see what I have painted and wrote about and say something that would just make all the agony seem it was for a purpose, and not just some fantasy that melted my mind. Most schizophrenics don't remember there psychosis, I on the other hand can tell you exactly where I went other than the times I was sleep walking through the streets of Vancouver. Sometimes even while I was on my medications, I felt from the heart that the music somehow called me to a place that was on the tip of my fingers. If I just could extend my arm a little more I would be able to grasp that place of being that was on the edge of awakening. The thoughts seemed to be making me clairvoyant and psychic. Are the thoughts I think my own or am I ultra-sensitive to other people's emotion and other people's thoughts. Where is that line I cross from being empathetic to psychotic? Sometimes my emotions are so great I try to form them to words like riddles and poems. Its tools like this that tell me understand who I am; it's like therapy to the soul. Is there a way to understand how another person feels through emotion? Of course but to understand that someone is going through a trauma of psychosis can be tough to figure out. Understanding schizophrenia takes a bit of empathy and insight to the person experiencing unusual thoughts or emotions. But it's strange fact that someone with unusual thoughts or emotions are passed off as eccentric. Which in a lot of cases most artists are, sometimes we fear ourselves as much as we fear love, if we face who we are then maybe we can face the things we love with honesty and joy and love in return. I am great full for understanding who I am, and who I love, even though what I love may be unattainable, I will always love it none the less without regret or shame.

It's ironic how similar love and schizophrenia is, in the

fact it can put you on the brink of reality, during my psychosis I did not feel Schizophrenic I felt in love to the point I felt fear. I felt if I followed love with the person who was utterly unattainable somehow it would be a reality but the reality I was following was a fantasy delusion. Where does one make sense of delusions of love and fantasy to illness and psychosis? I think the part that defines love is that no matter how much you want it you have to be at peace with letting it come and go as it chooses. We are not in control of love the control is an illusion. Love just is what it is nothing more. And it is always free. That's where my romantic side kicks in; by some act of fate will Sandra read between the lines, will she read what I have written? Will our paths cross? I am willing to say no it won't yet at the same time I think of what a romance it would be to never meet her in my lifetime and to tell her in the afterlife where I took what I had, and there the Truth would be known of how I felt all along. The love letter suicide note, interesting who the two could be taken for one or the other, yet I could never bring myself to end my life. I would live to as long as was meant for me to carry what I have to the bitter end of time before I would ever consider that. For me I will never die, in my eyes the dance of life and death as always present. And even though this may sound like poetry of an ill-fated man. I am proud to have at least sparked the fire. I hope that someday people will consider that we are human too, and not the monsters that the stigma makes use out to be. One thing that I do know is that for whatever reason this was my gift not a curse to share with people. I hope that people will understand what insight I could give. peoples aunts uncles mother fathers brothers and sisters are all capable of falling to schizophrenia, I hope in some way the shadow to their nightmare for you the ones who are not sick can understand that we need you to be loving to the people, not monsters, or irrational members of your family. Without you, we would be lost. Without my family I probably would have taken a lot longer to recover if at all. It may seem like a roller coaster at first but it is possible for someone to become stable to the point they are almost fully recovered. Compassion and insight makes the process a lot easier because without compassion or insight, there would only be darkness. Family was what kept me from dying so did Sandra so I guess I did have more than one angel on my side, I had many, even my friends helped. When I went missing they went looking for me, when I was admitted to one south they were there to help me through it. They gave me the courage to accept that something in fact was not right. In my mind were ghosts, but in the world around me was not what I was thinking. Taking a long time to decipher between the two was an on-going process that if I did not have my family and friends, I would have been on the streets for the rest of my life. there's a lot of things that come to mind when people think of the word Schizophrenia, a lot of negative words, it's ironic that the voices we here are negative as well, but who do we believe the voices in our heads or what society or other people view us as. all those negative thoughts that other people have about schizophrenia is 1% true, that leaves a lot of us who have not given the VOICE we need to tell other people that we ARE NOT all killers and mass murderers. it's time that we stop listening to the negativity that popular media portrays us as and that we start to accept people with any type of mental illness beautiful gifted human beings. Maybe what I'm trying to say is as much of a dream as having Sandra as a friend, as a mutual inspired muse. Maybe all this is something that will never be or whispers lost in the nights wind. The duality I face of poetry and logic are something of a moonlight dance. Where my logic is on my left hand and my poetry artistic is on my right, as if I was wired differently than most human beings. Society puts us in separate categories and yet we feel inhuman towards ourselves in our own minds, where do we find out that we are human like everyone else? If I could say to people look if you cut me do I not bleed? The scholar in me comes forth when I wish to portray another light into the mind of who I am. I love life I love being on this earth I hope I can out live anyone. I wish for eternal life. For the longer I live the more wisdom attains. Recently I have been seeing a new psychiatrist, to be reassessed. Things are good they now have medications that don't have the horrible side effects of diabetes, weight gain, and high cholesterol. I have been off Risperdal for a few weeks now and switched to ability. For me I felt more psychotic on Risperdal and more human on ability. I've lost weight and I am starting to gain my self-esteem back. The process is still on-going but every day I am proud of who I am and what I went through. I am gracious to be alive. And no matter what I will always listen to the music that inspires me. Who is the man in the chair I talked about, it was me I had a vision that I would be forever in a chair until the new age. Well I have been working on computers ever since I was diagnosed sitting in front playing games to keep me active. I guess that vision was not so far off. I also predicted I would go missing of four days in my journal. Did I somehow know what would happen to me in the future? Was I somehow living a prophecy? Do I somehow feel I will be among stars that shine oh so bright? To me life is the romantic journey of a dance of light and love. Where my road leads I do not know, but somehow I hear the singing, that follows me so. Do I love her? I do not know. Do I admire her, always? I guess one could say in a crowded room I'm the one in the corner, looking at a distance through the white padded walls. With little windows I write on the walls and a door that has no handle. I walk to my pedestal from a dull glow of the moon through the window. And reflecting love to the one beside me. I do not need to look at her beauty fills me so. The love I feel is true but the dream I'm in is my reality. If I were to say I love her dearly, it would only fall as rain to the soil below. Leave tears for the tree among a fairy tales glow, and I whisper a lullaby in the night sleep tight in a whimsical snow. It all seems so real yet what I can't understand is why me why did I have to endure something that my mind made up or rather that I fell into like a rabbit hole. The parallels to Alice in wonderland seem a bit forthcoming. In my lifetime I hope that people with my illness are not met with fear or something to be swept under the rug. I hope that more people come to realize that not everyone with schizophrenia becomes lost for a lifetime that in fact with proper support anyone with the illness can recover. My hopes and dreams from logic are so much different than my hopes and dreams of the artist. Part of me wants to break down what I am and the other part of me wants to express who I am. Duality presents itself in the face of the love that I so fear, and yet I know that facing my fear I can learn to love without conditions. If my eyes told the story would sand be able to see it from looking into them. The fear of looking her in the eyes would overwhelm me. Yet longing for her to be in my arms would be so humbling I would melt and melt and melt as ice to the light of the sun. Her words sauce my soul and to create something from the whispers of the voice that pulls my heart is like a drug in the night. Being an icon to someone who has nothing but a few belongings seems so distant, yet the hope one day the diamond in the rough is known to the world as someone to be cherished as a person to come back from the brink of hell would be quite amazing. that's what it's all about after all isn't, having the courage to come back from the darkest places of hell and return to the living and embracing life? In so many ways I want to have that bit of acknowledgement to make the time in my own purgatory have some sort of justification. To have an ending where the guy does in fact get the girl, after all a true romance never ends without a union of some kind. But is this romance truly over will fate drive together what seems to be impossible? I truly hope so, because it would take a miracle in my own humble opinion. Who is Sandra? She is a ghost, an angel, a muse. My unattainable love who I wait for on the pedestal in my tower. The writings on the walls travel to different rooms with windows to the moon, and I forever look upon the moonlight with fondness. In a lot of ways I feel the tower I live in is unbreakable, like the rook in an endless chess game. And in eternity the game over white and darkness is the universes duality in expanding and contracting. For I too feel endlessly small and endlessly large. With my own two feet I dance the dance and walk the walk until the sun sets on the tower I fall. I brew some coffee I light a smoke and this is now my addictions. They are unbreakable and they are tools to cope. Without them I would really need to be in a padded white wall room. I am but one of many a light that shines I feel the love I hate the pain. In riddles I talk in morning you sang. May there be a person who understands that sometimes the words of someone who believes in love gets confused with the logic of stern rules. That love is to be contained as an object however ironic that is, it can break the largest rock and melt the coldest ice. If life is a game then winning is surviving life. but if you find the reason I should not be here, then you do not know what it means to be human, but that's a feeling I have when I think how lucky other people are who do not have health issues, is the grass greener on the other side of the fence? I say don't judge a man until you have walked a mile in their shoes. And sometimes those shoes are pretty worn out from the endless walking down dark and lonely roads. If there was a time to embrace people with mental illness like Schizophrenia, it's now. It's time for the world to wake up and accept that we are human too. One day the things in my mind will make sense and one day my love will be real. I did have a dream though. I would see myself years from now older 50's flying in my personal jet; I became a writer and an advocate. The cause was something no one wanted to deal with, something that everyone tried to keep under the carpet. I take the fight of the stigma of mental illness and Schizophrenia; I raise the flag of awareness, and March towards the front lines. No one really knows what the term schizophrenia meant. Hell I still don't even know. All I know is it's a label that judges. If I had to use my face to put to the label I would, and if I ever win a Nobel prize for being a writer.....Well a man can dream cant he?........